A View from the Head End

Medical cartoons to ease the pain

By Steve Yentis

tfm Publishing Ltd, Castle Hill Barns, Harley, Nr Shrewsbury, SY5 6LX, UK.
Tel: +44 (0)1952 510061; Fax: +44 (0)1952 510192
E-mail: nikki@tfmpublishing.com; Web site: www.tfmpublishing.com

Design and type-setting: Nikki Bramhill

ISBN 1 903378 42 7

Printed by Gutenberg Press Ltd., Gudja Road, Tarxien, PLA 19, Malta.
Tel: +356 21897037; Fax: +356 21800069.

Contents

		Page
Foreword		iv
Chapter 1.	The wards zone	1
Chapter 2.	Counting backwards	11
Chapter 3.	Theatricals	16
Chapter 4.	Expensive scare	34
Chapter 5.	State of the art	39
Chapter 6.	Counting on colleagues	51
Chapter 7.	Mothers and babies	59
Chapter 8.	Special occasions	72
Chapter 9.	The boundaries of knowledge	78
Chapter 10.	Painful clinics	86
Chapter 11.	Passing the exam	92
Chapter 12.	Pot-pourri	109

Foreword

Most of the following collection has been drawn between cases, before (and occasionally during) meetings, and at odd moments snatched between various duties and activities during the last couple of decades. Most, but not all, are anaesthetic in nature. Some were for posters, some for slide presentations, some for specific publications, but most were just for fun. The materials range from artists' pens to NHS ballpoints, and from proper drawing paper, through various non-vital portions of patients' notes, to the back of surgical glove wrappers - hence the sometimes rushed appearance and frankly, poor artwork. To preserve the spirit of the moment in which they were drawn, and to avoid any extra work for the humble artist, the cartoons have been left in their original state, complete with wonky headings and captions. I still hope they entertain, or at least strike a chord.

Steve M Yentis

June 2005

Acknowledgement

The cartoons on pages 94, 96, 99, 101 and 105 have been reproduced with permission from Elsevier, ©2002. R Sharpe, M Brunner, S Yentis, M Hasan, N Robinson. *The Primary FRCA: A Complete Guide to Preparation and Passing*. Butterworth-Heinemann, 2002: pp 8, 20, 144, 227, 290.

The cartoons on pages 93, 95, 97, 98, 100, 102, 103, 104, 107 and 108 have been reproduced with permission from Elsevier. © 1998 SM Yentis. SM Yentis. *FRCA Survival Guide*. Butterworth-Heinemann, 1998: pp 5, 60, 38, 36, 62, 75, 79, 90, 88, 92.

Chapter 1

The wards zone

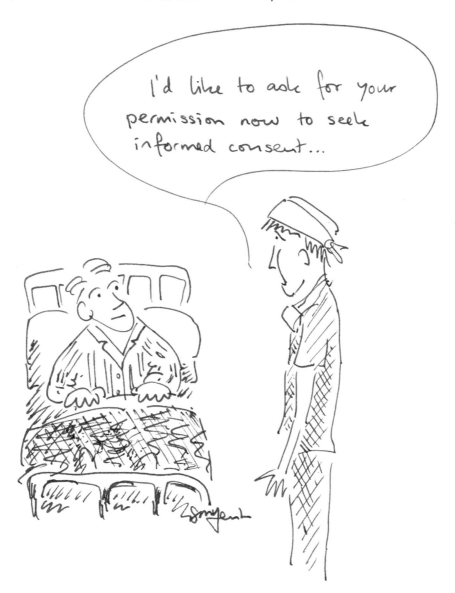

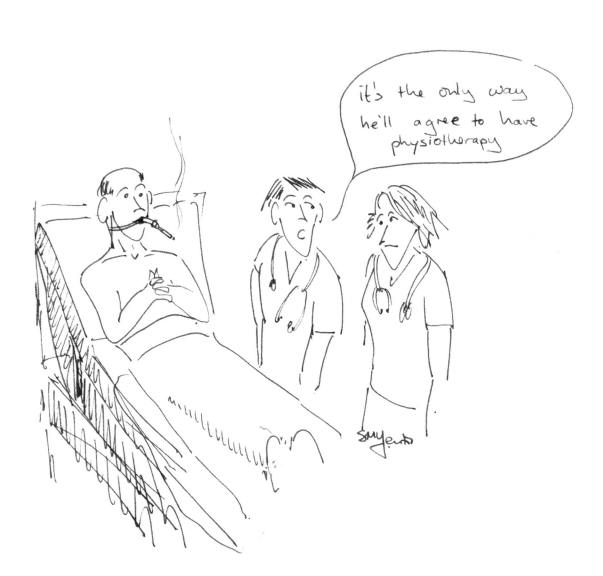

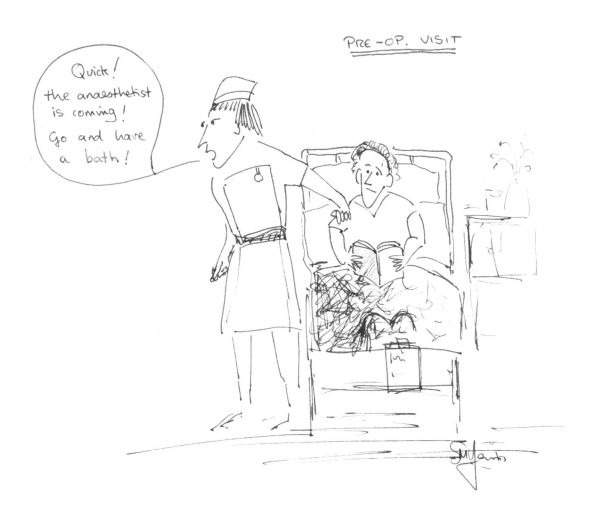

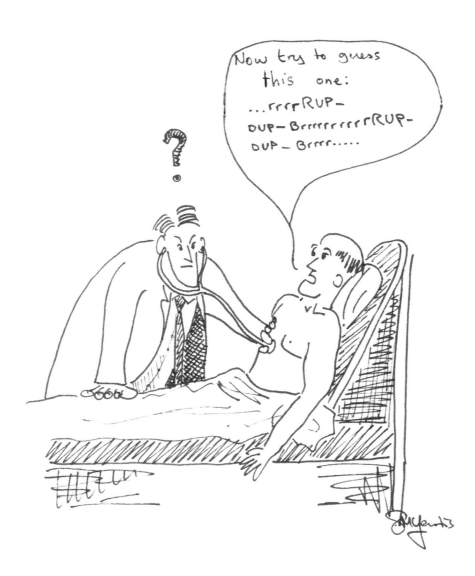

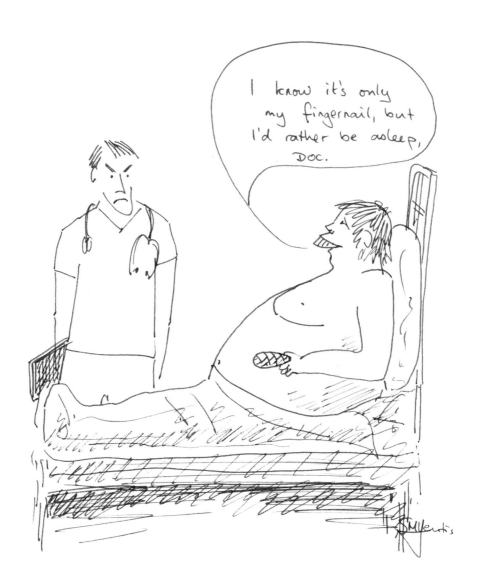

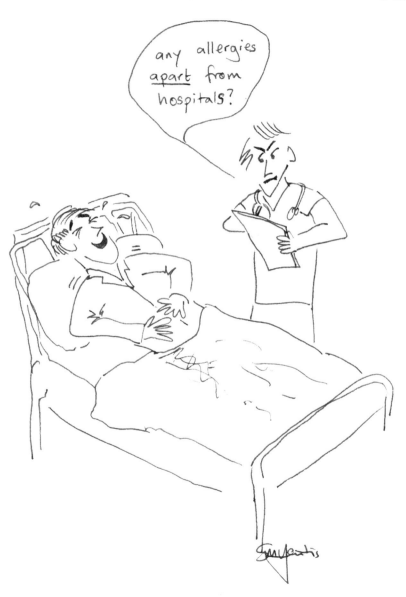

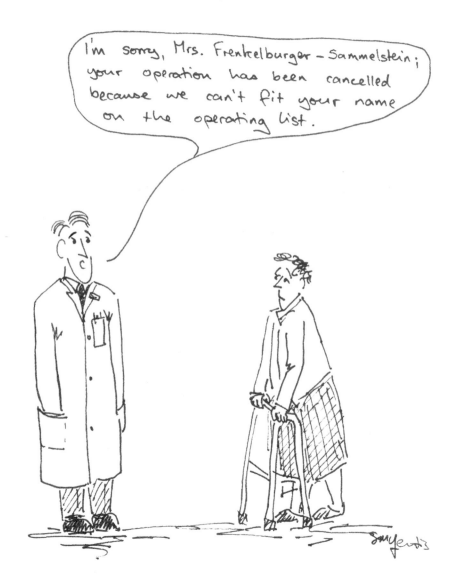

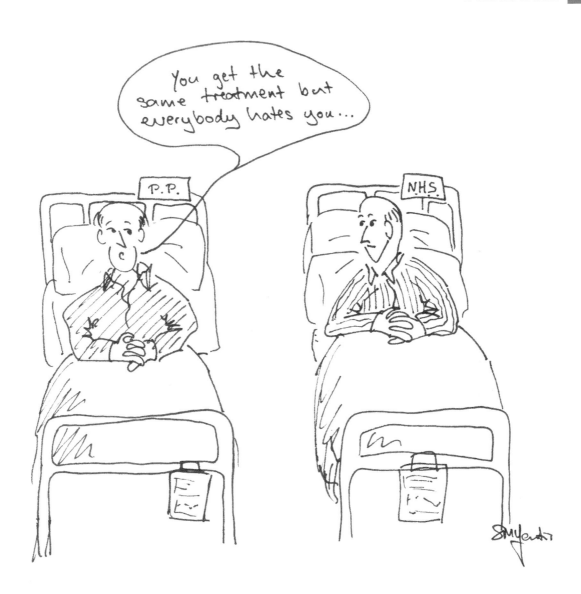

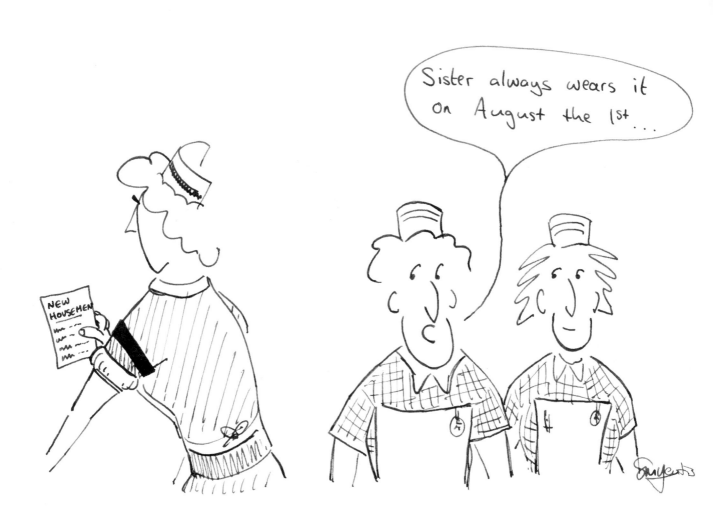

Chapter 2

Counting backwards

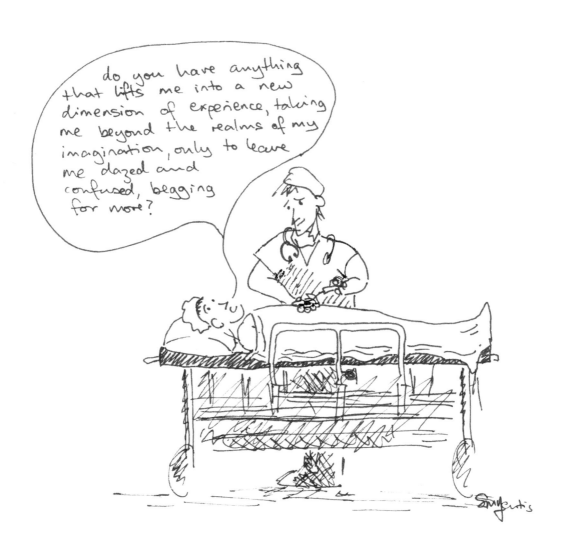

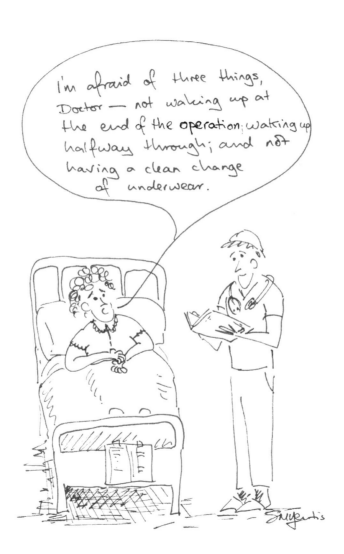

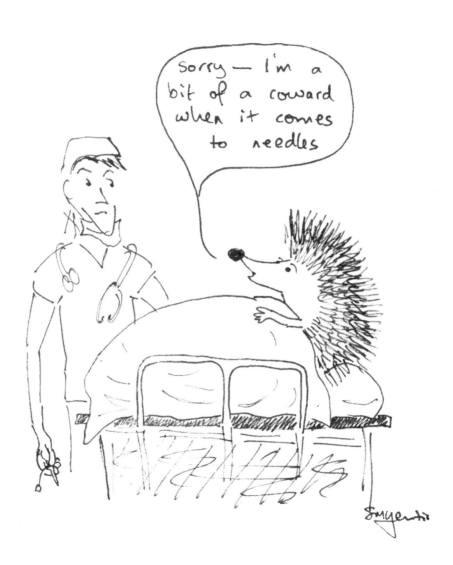

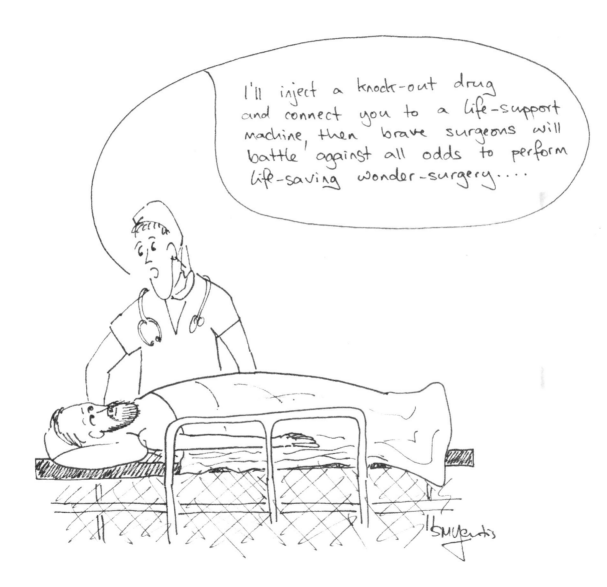

Chapter 3

Theatricals

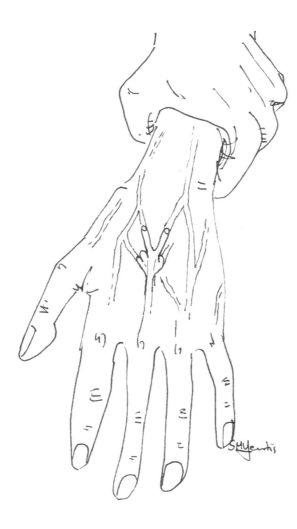

LOOKING FOR A VEIN

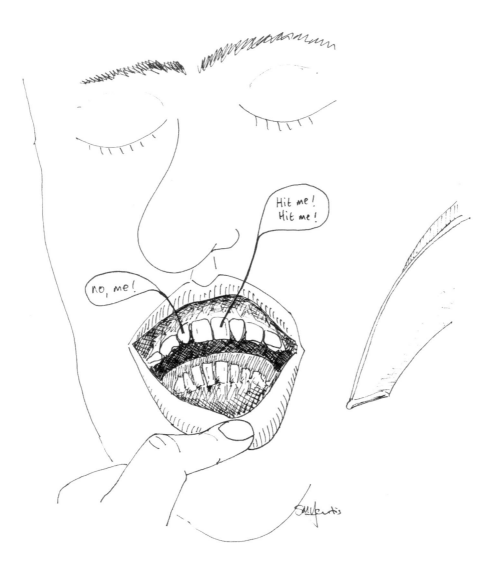

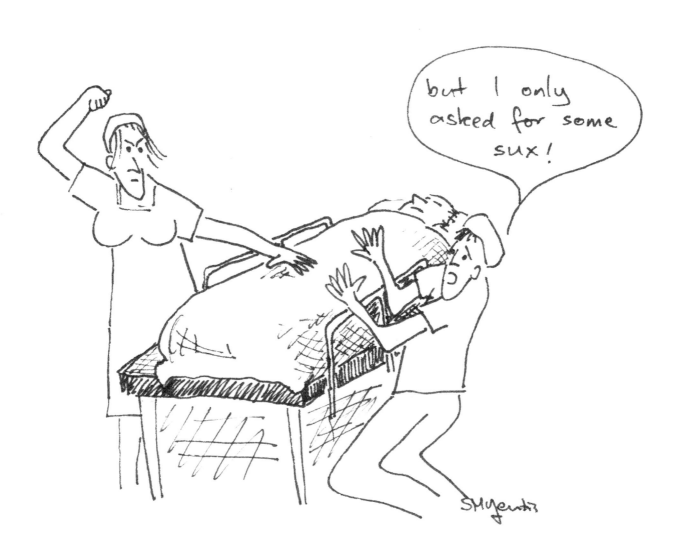

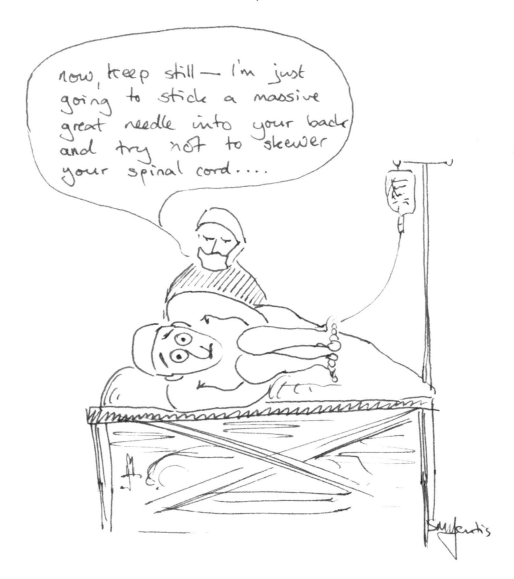

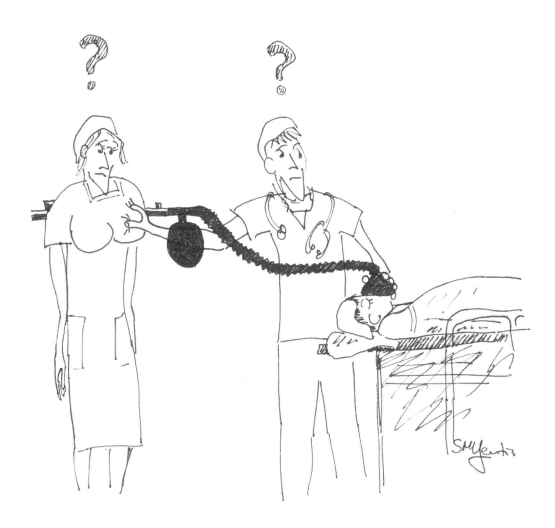

THE OBESE PATIENT.

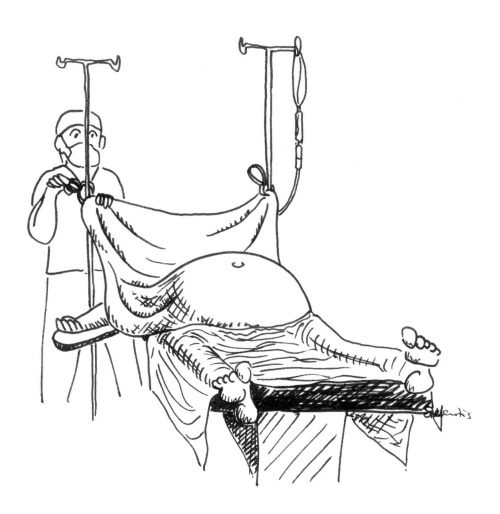

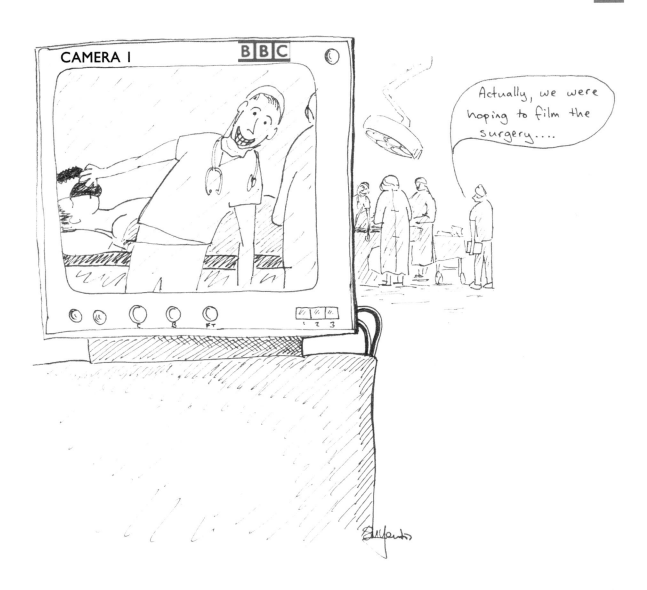

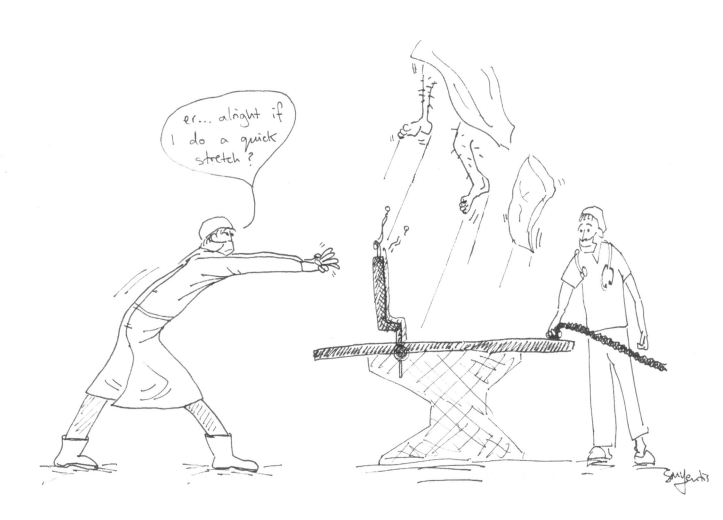

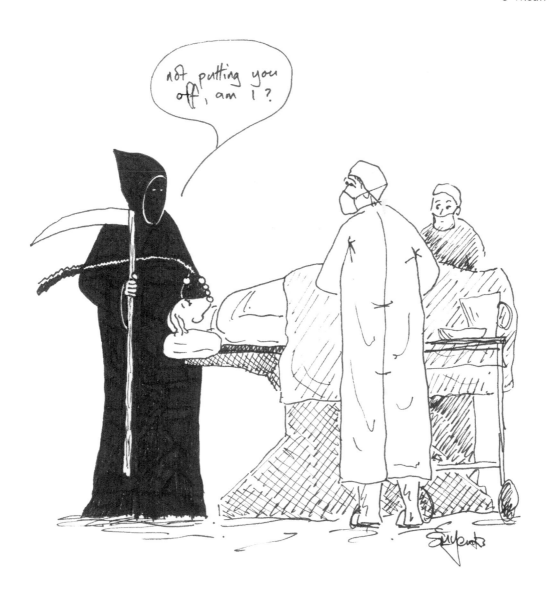

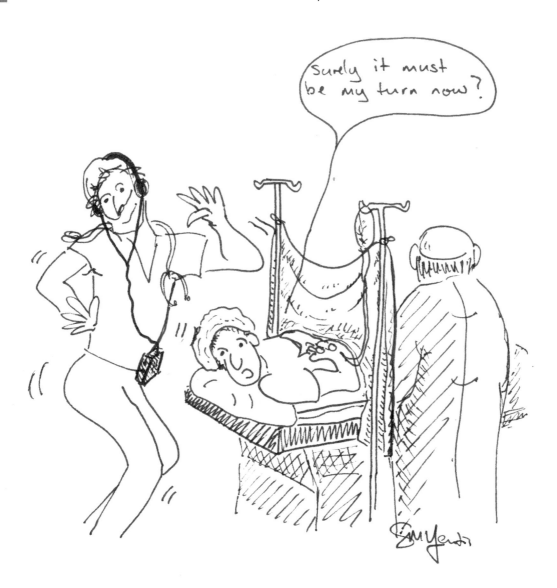

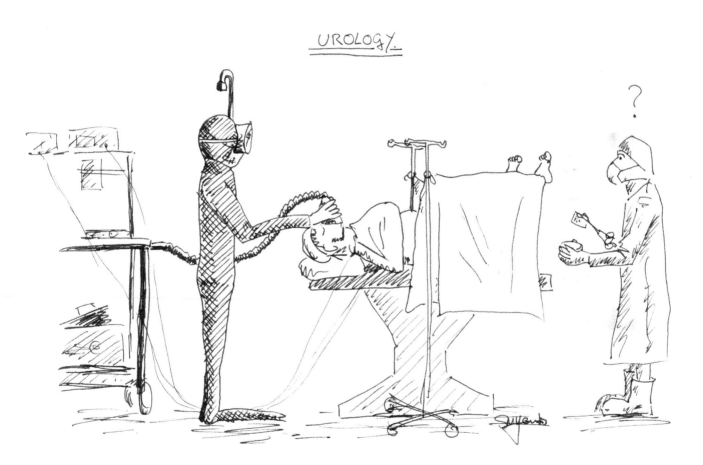

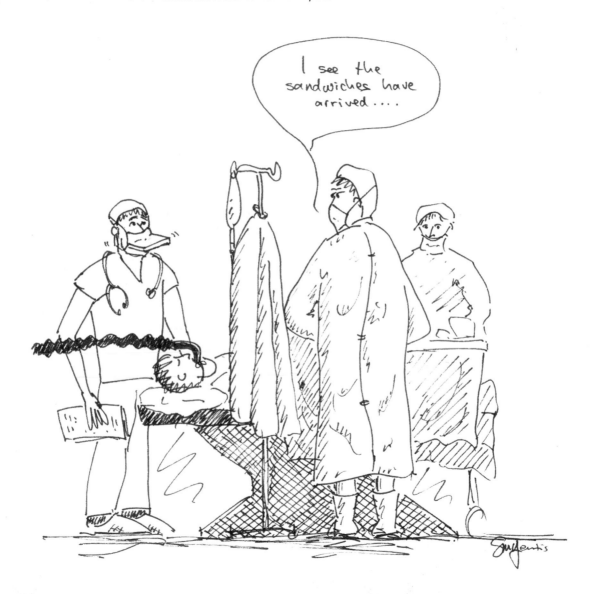

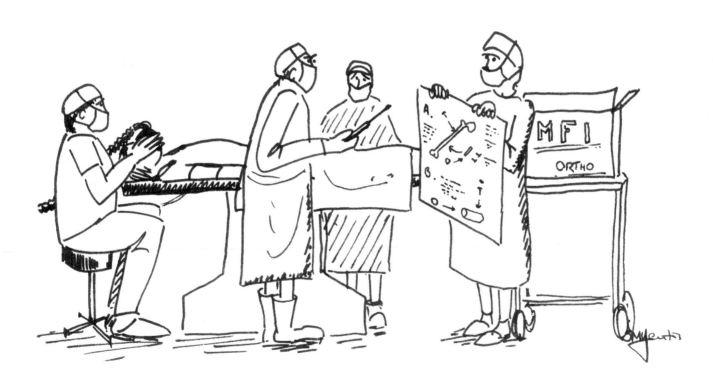

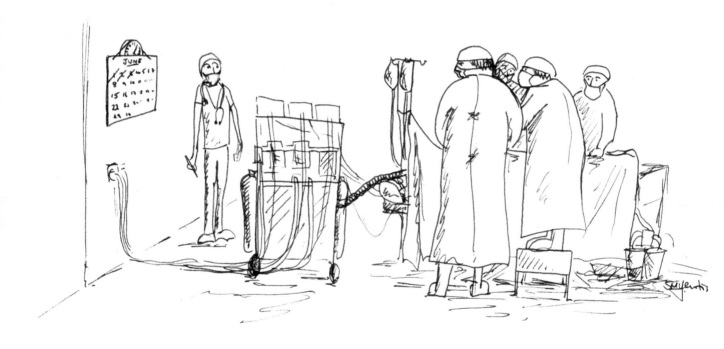

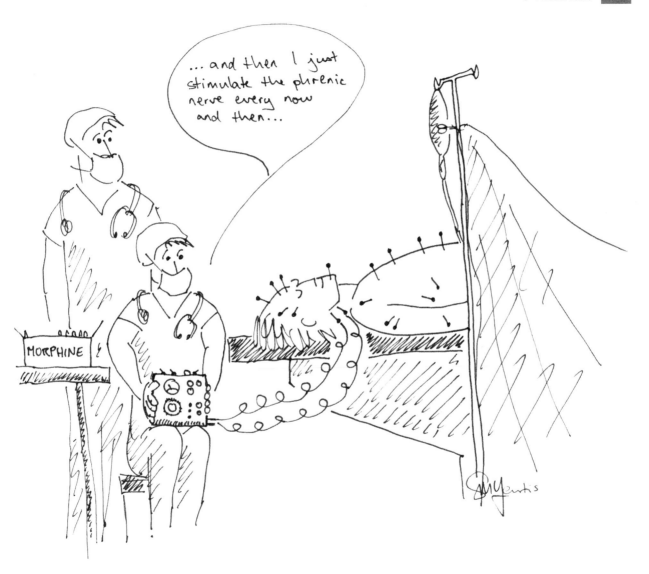

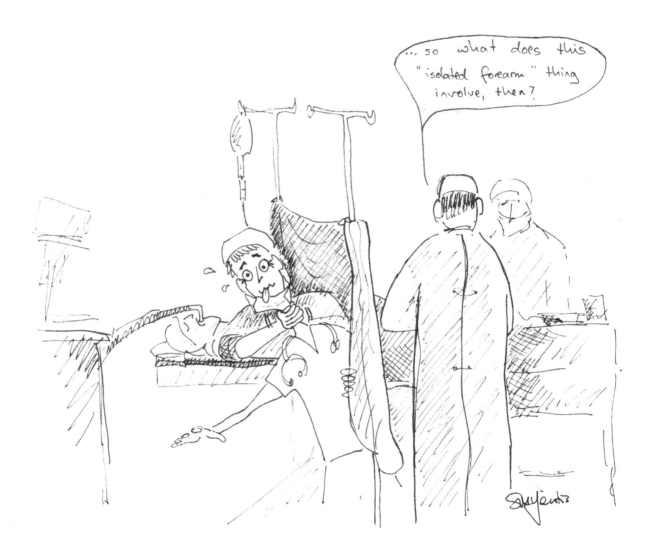

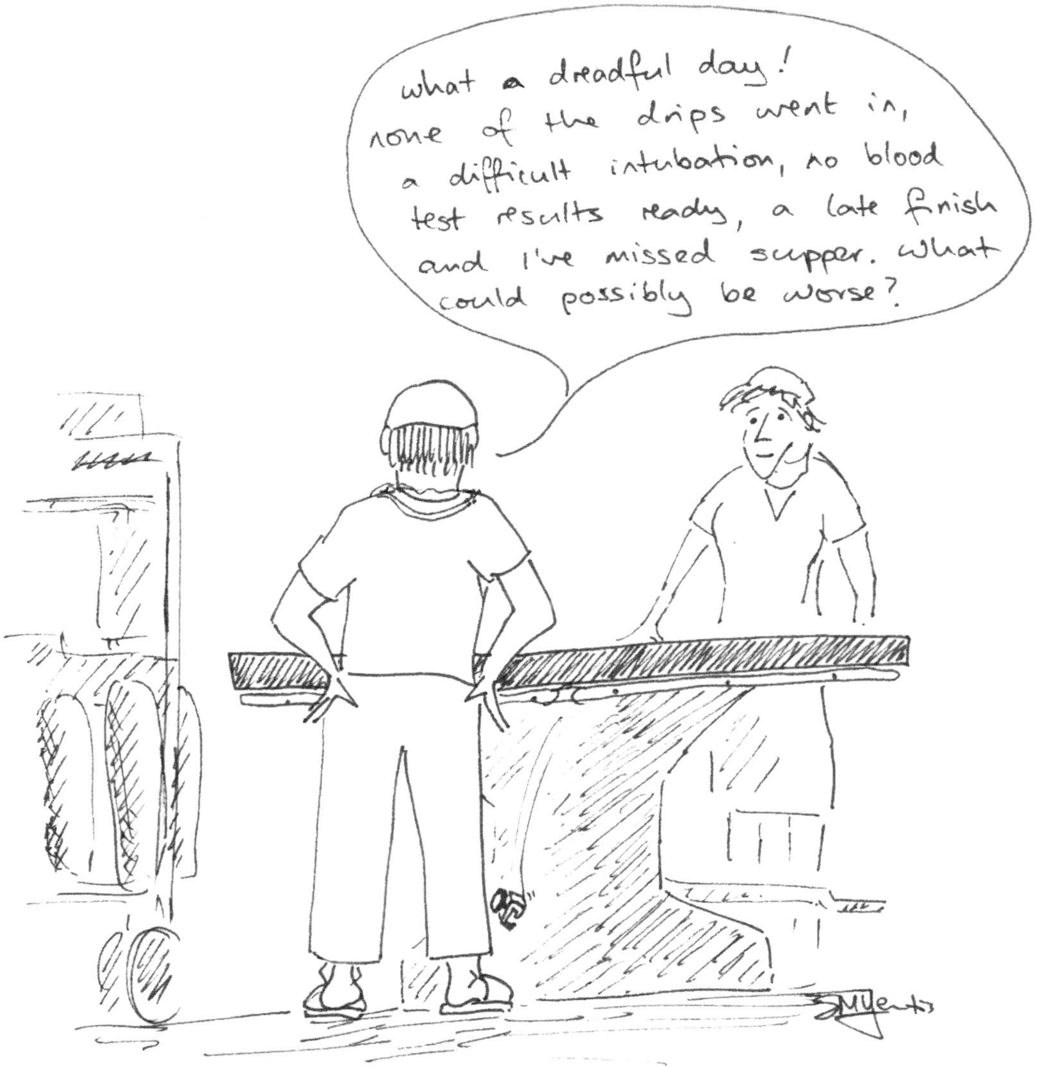
what a dreadful day! none of the drips went in, a difficult intubation, no blood test results ready, a late finish and I've missed supper. What could possibly be worse?
SMYeats

Chapter 4

Expensive scare

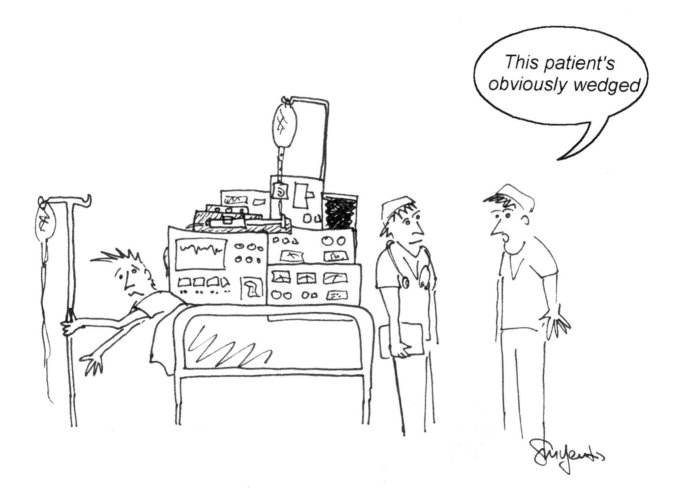

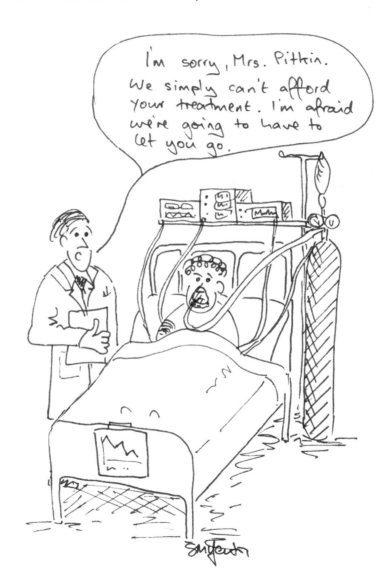

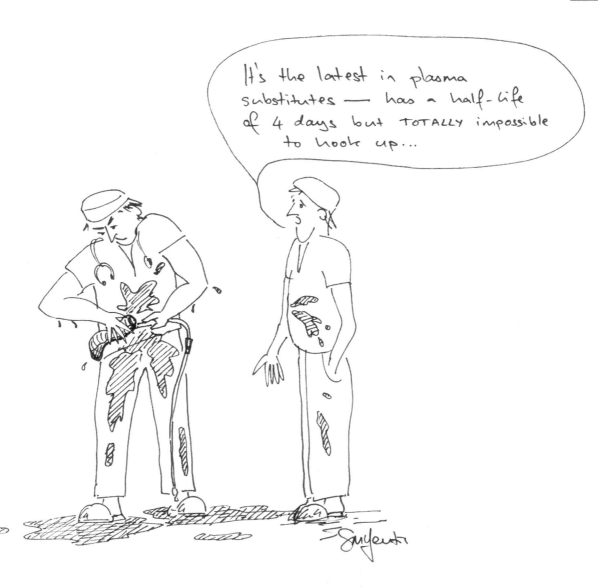

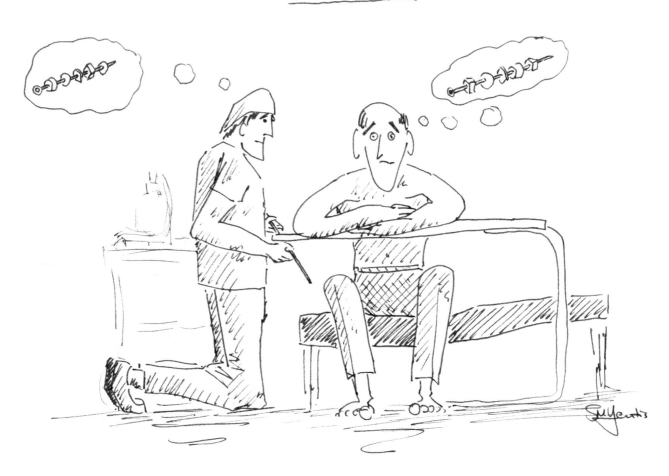

Chapter 5

State of the art

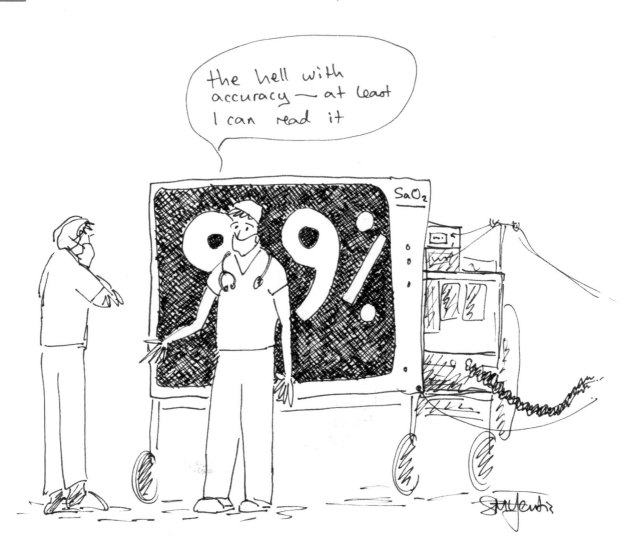

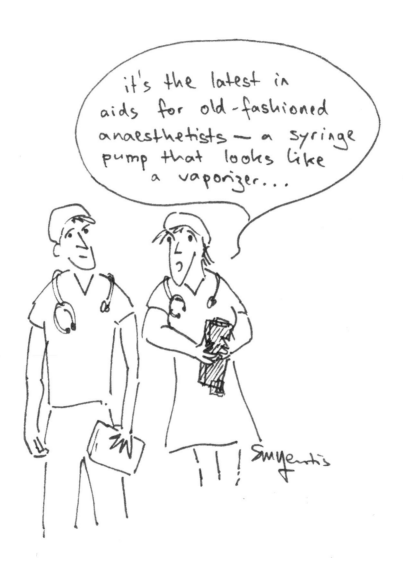

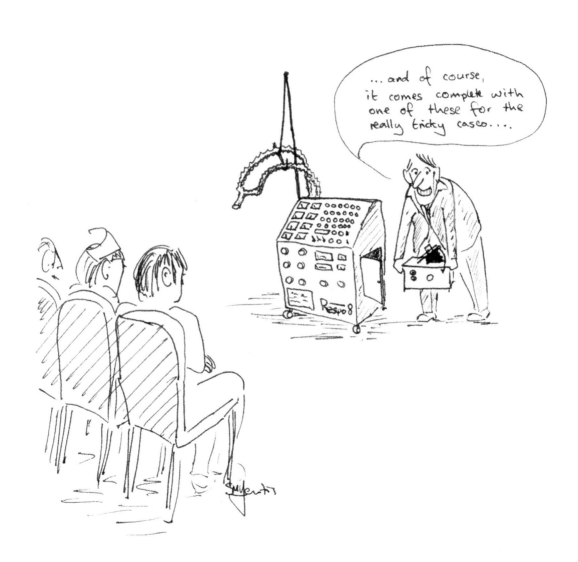

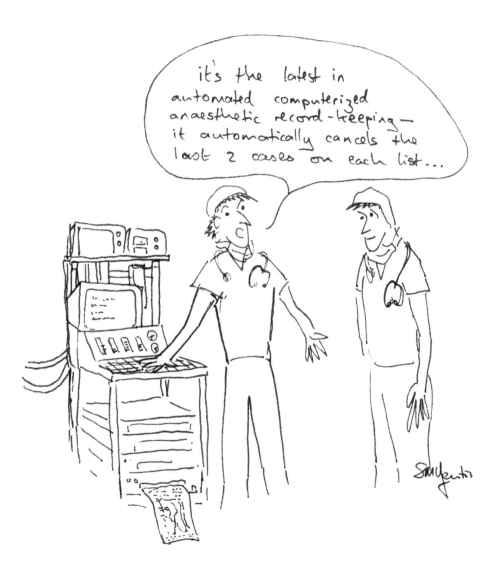

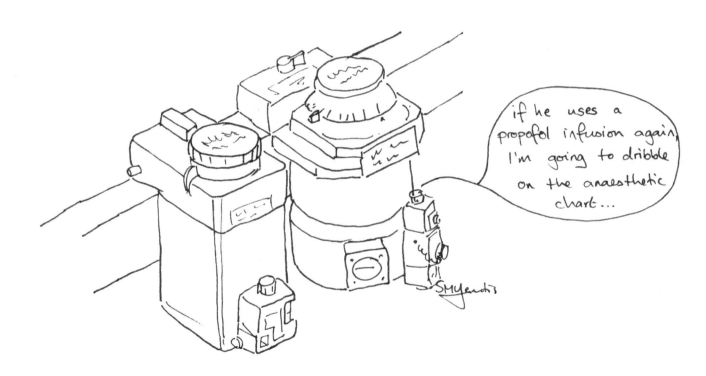

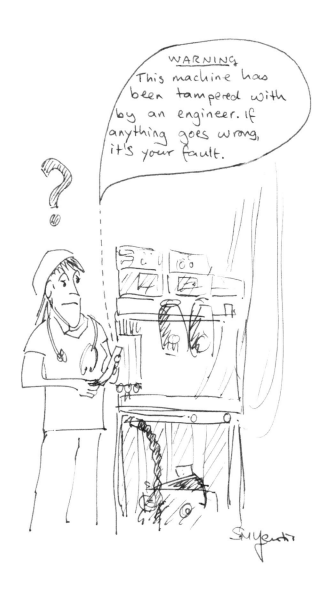

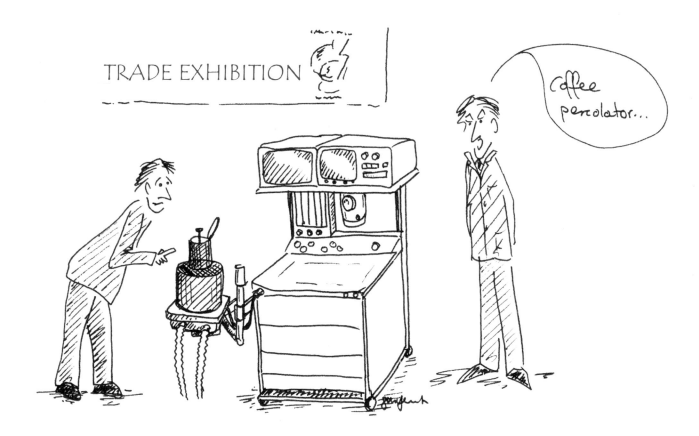

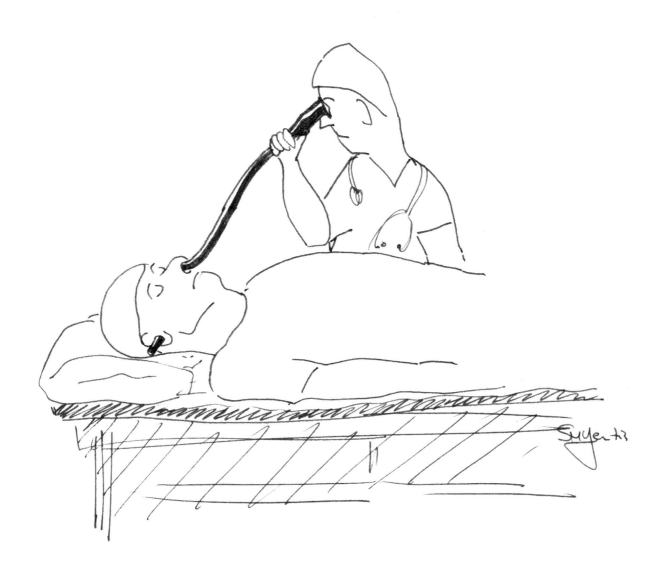

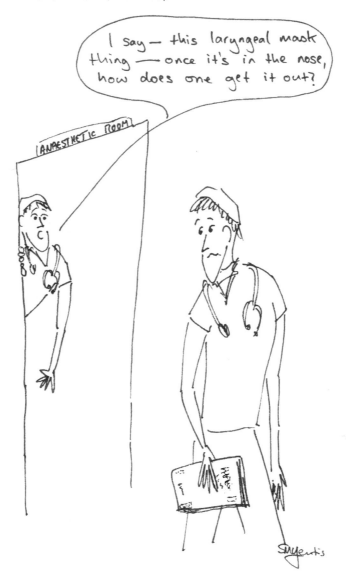

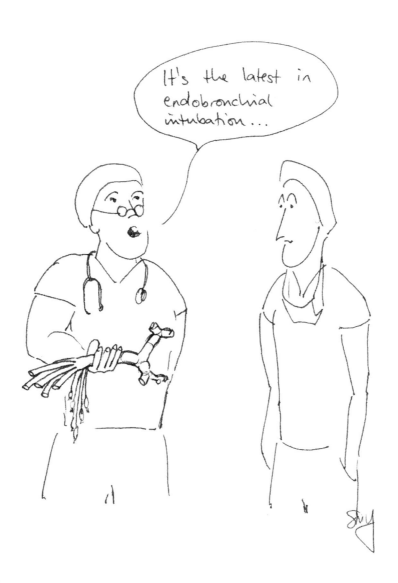

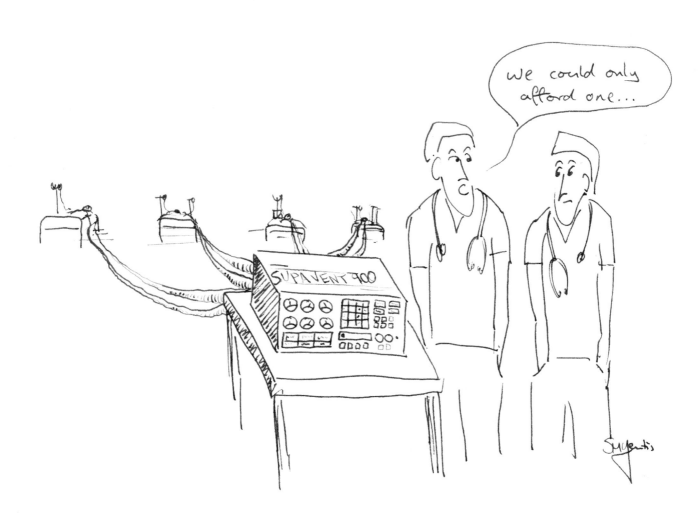

Chapter 6

Counting on colleagues

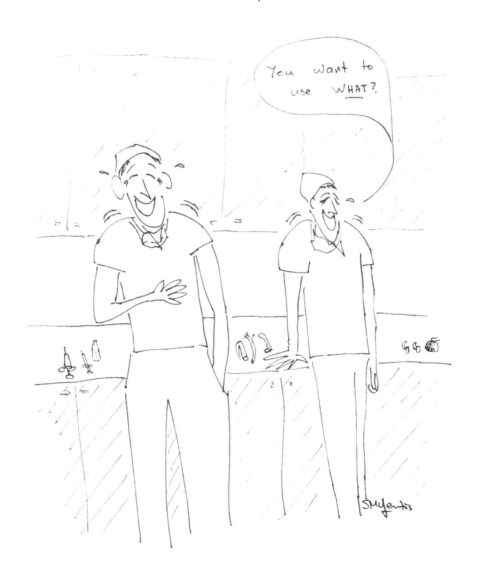

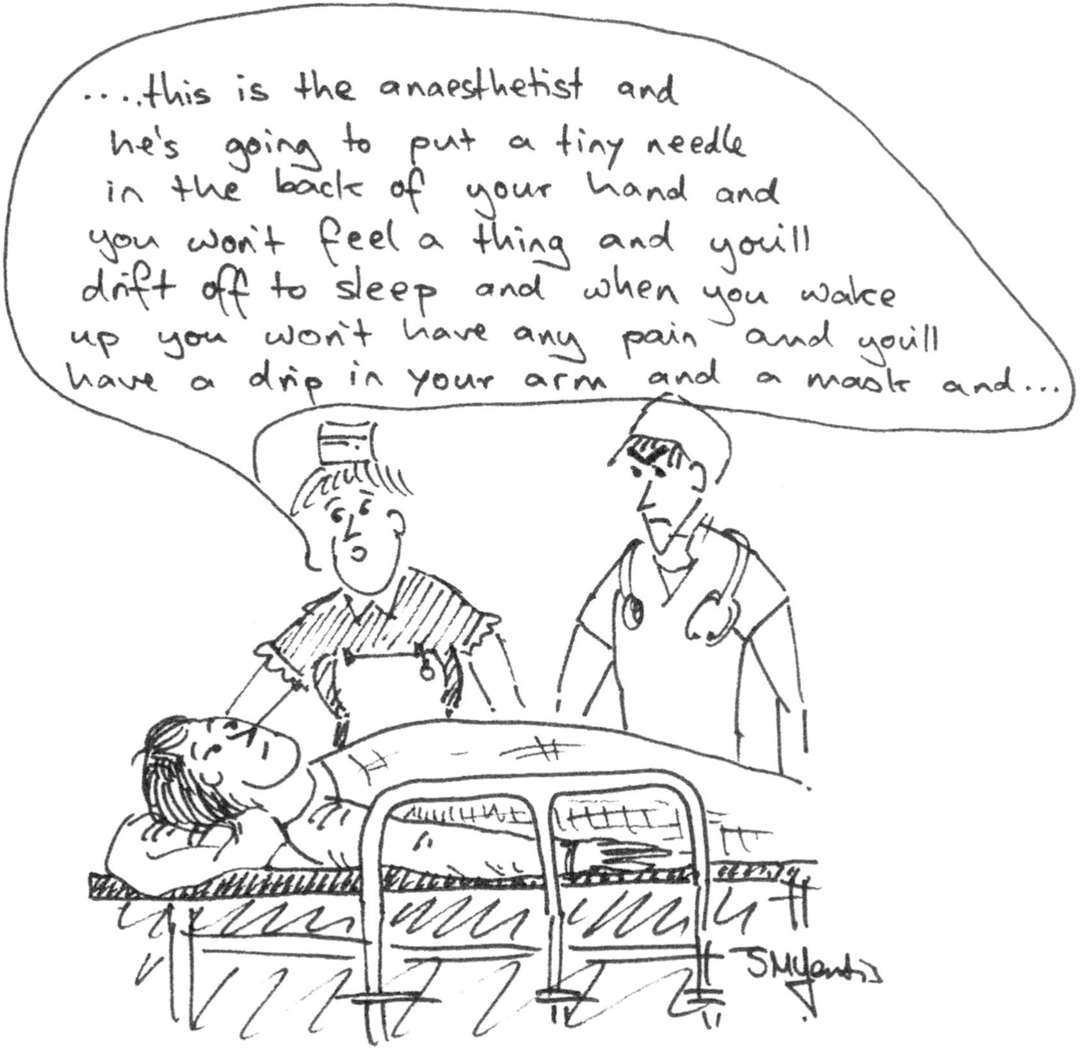
....this is the anaesthetist and he's going to put a tiny needle in the back of your hand and you won't feel a thing and you'll drift off to sleep and when you wake up you won't have any pain and you'll have a drip in your arm and a mask and...
SMYenti?

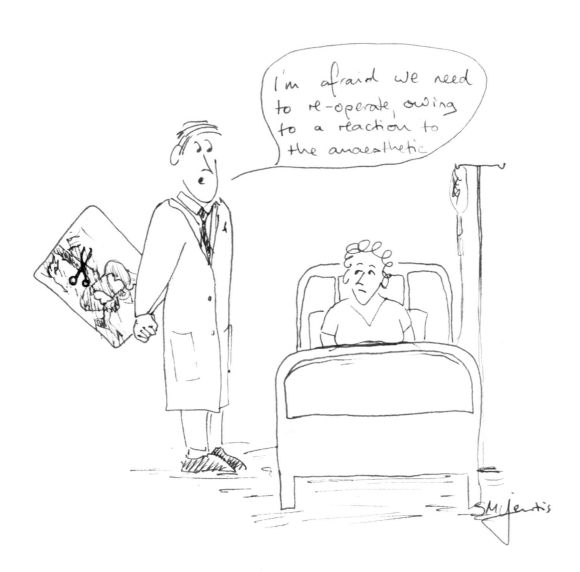

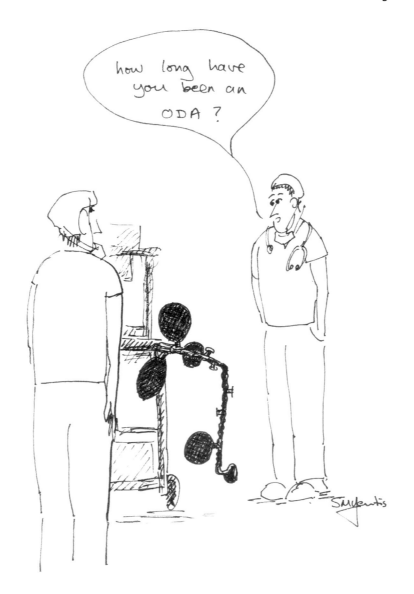

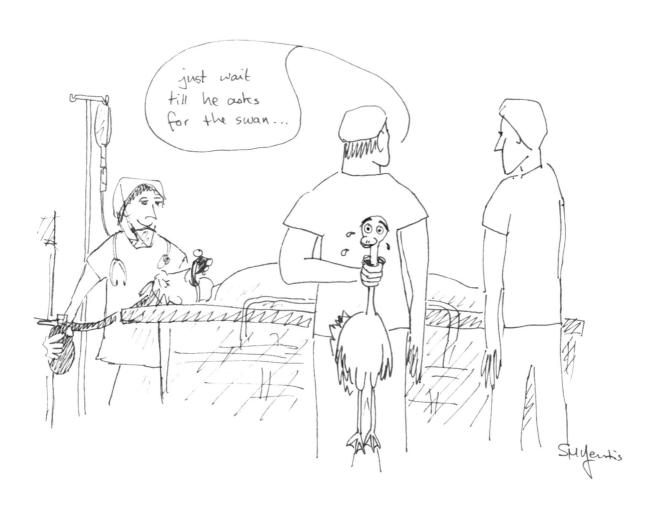

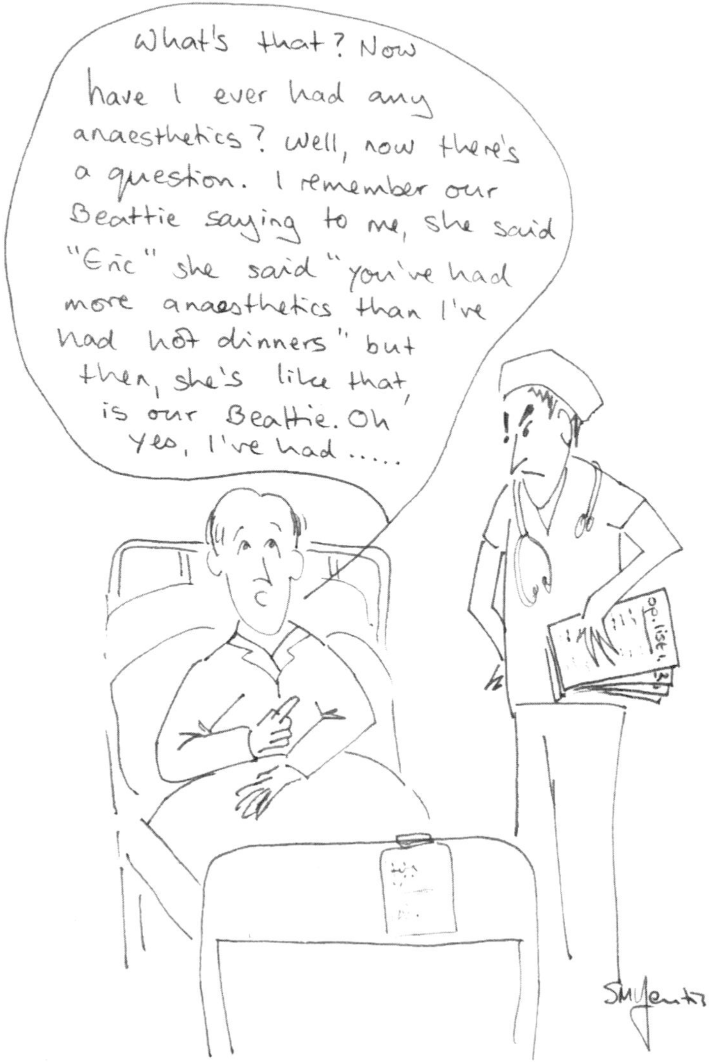
What's that? Now have I ever had any anaesthetics? Well, now there's a question. I remember our Beattie saying to me, she said "Eric" she said "you've had more anaesthetics than I've had hot dinners" but then, she's like that, is our Beattie. Oh yes, I've had .....
op. list

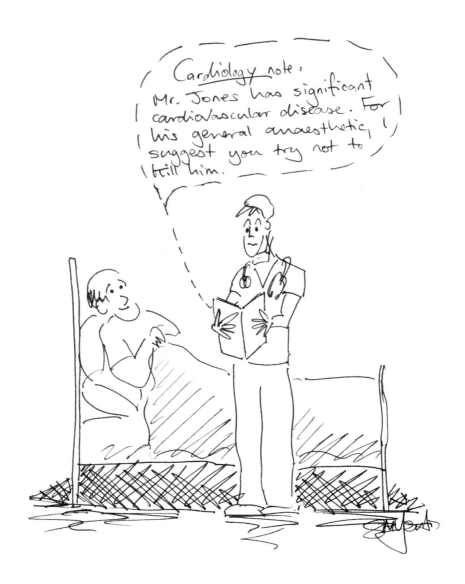

Chapter 7

Mothers and babies

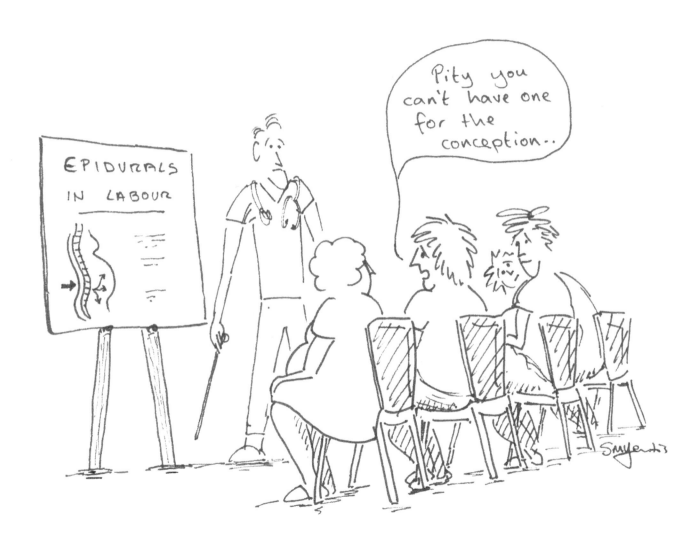

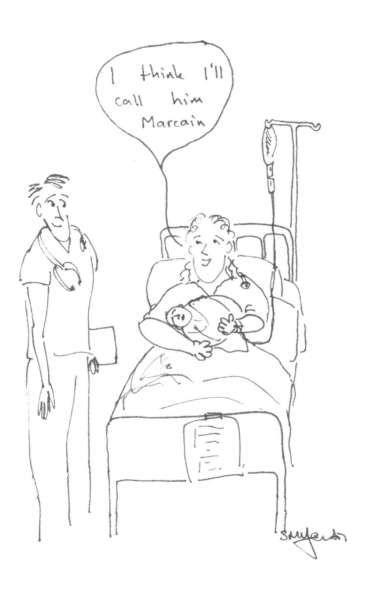

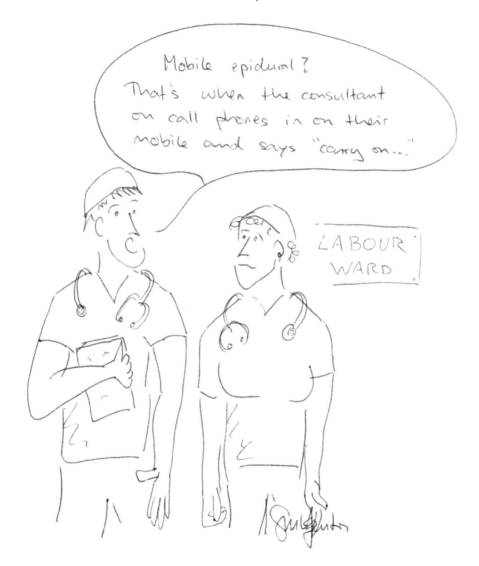

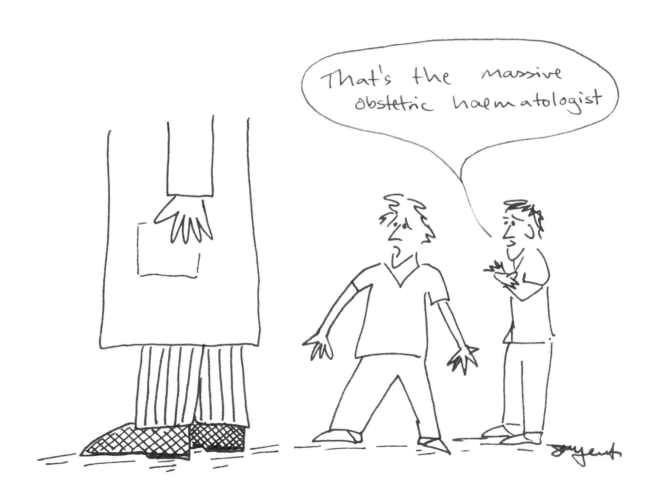

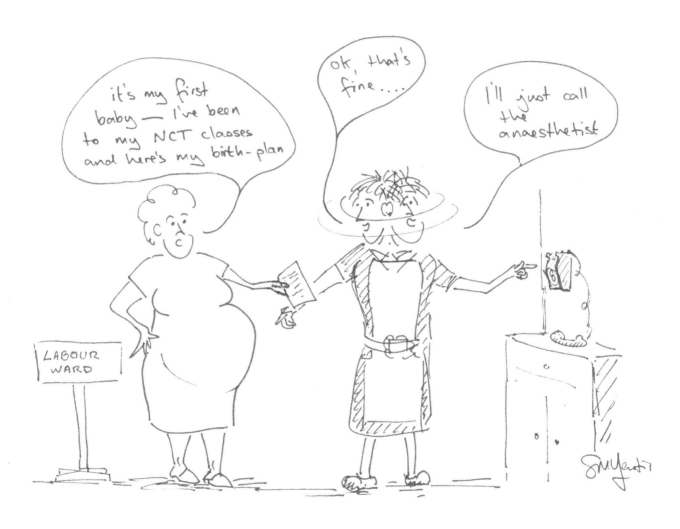

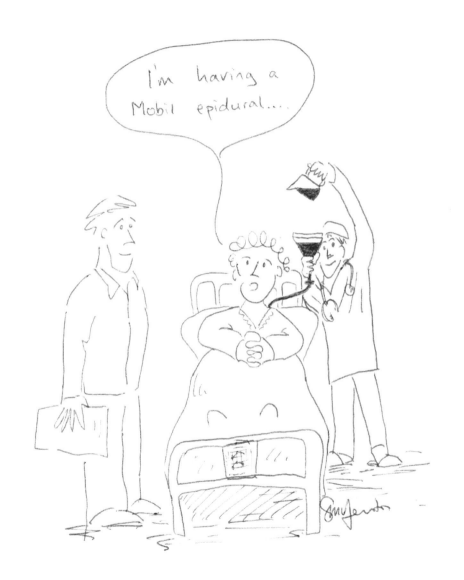

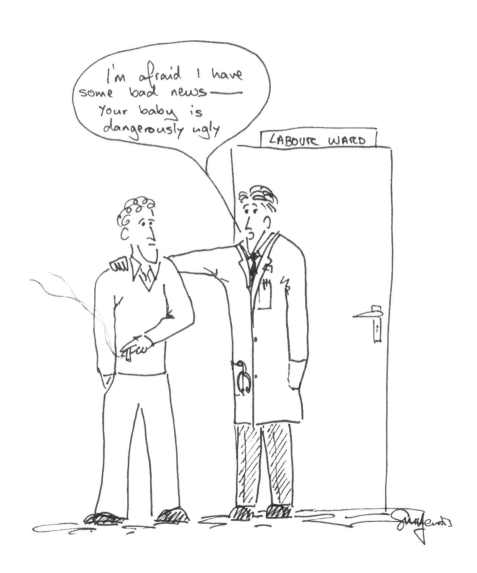

THE EFFECTS OF DRUGS ON THE NEWBORN

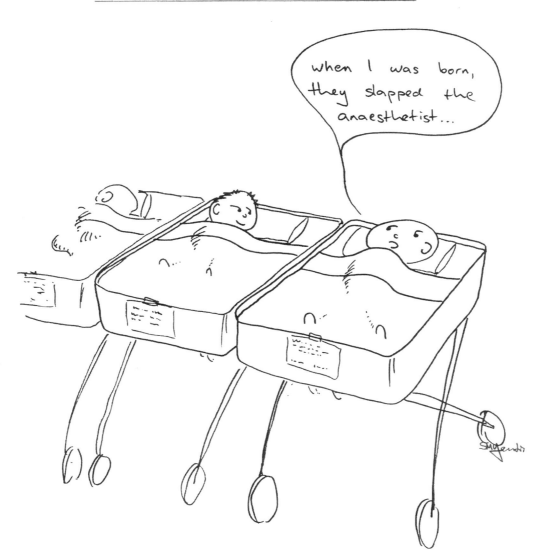

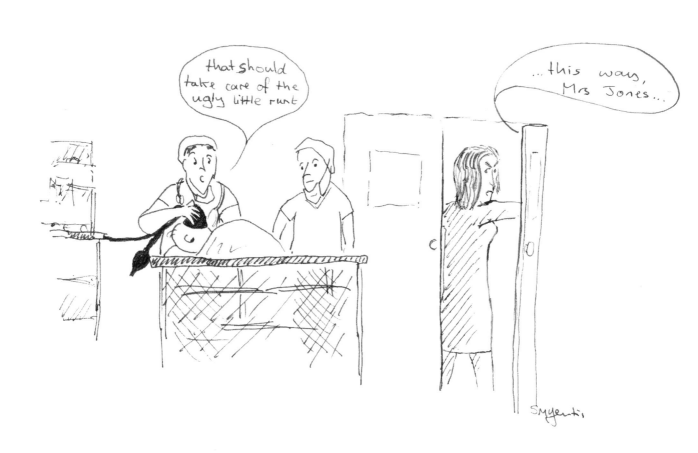

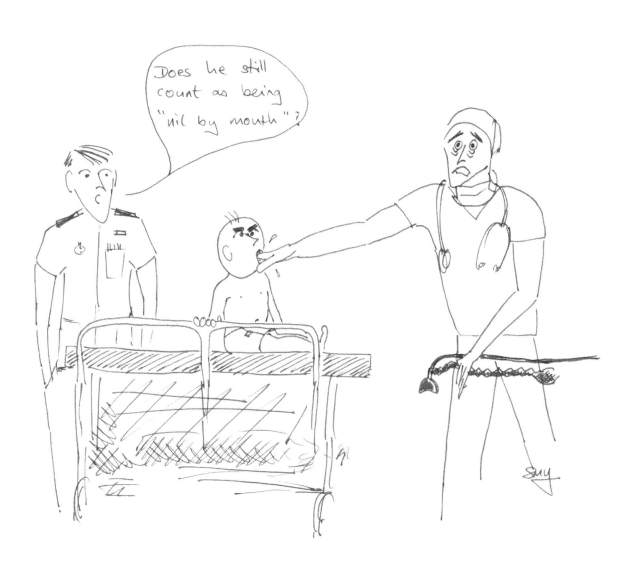

THE NEW SHO

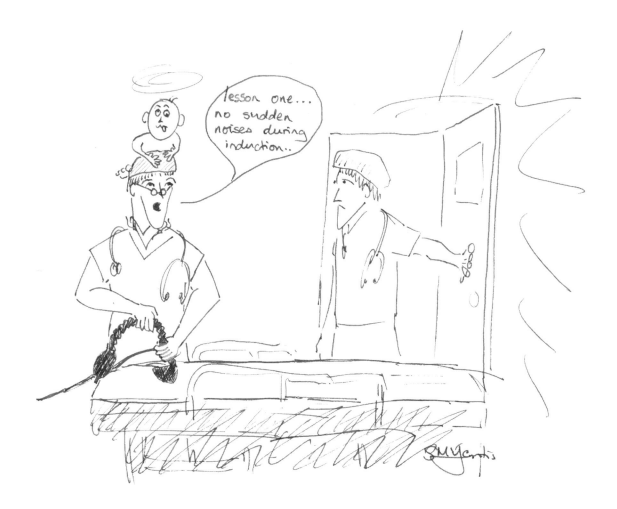

PAEDIATRIC INDUCTION

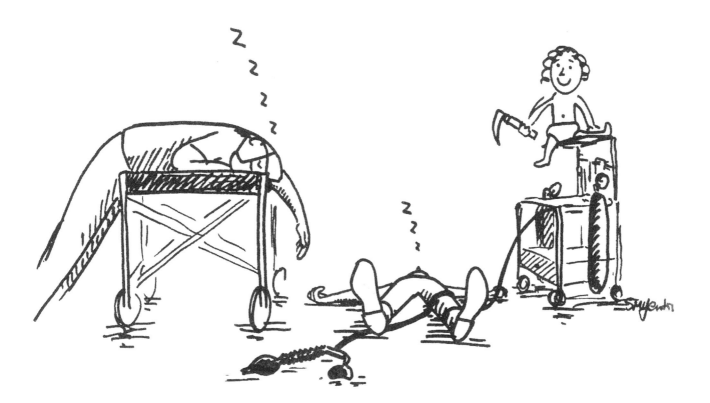

Chapter 8

Special occasions

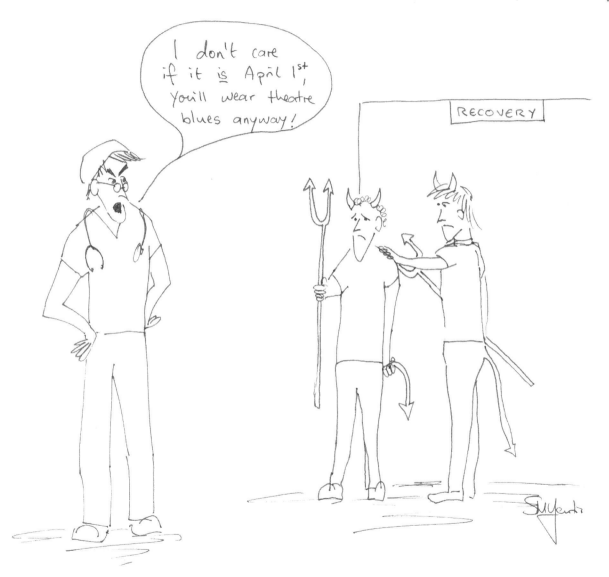

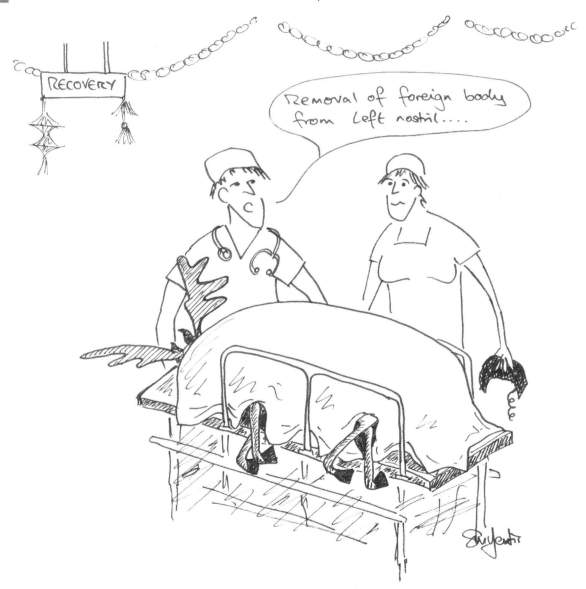

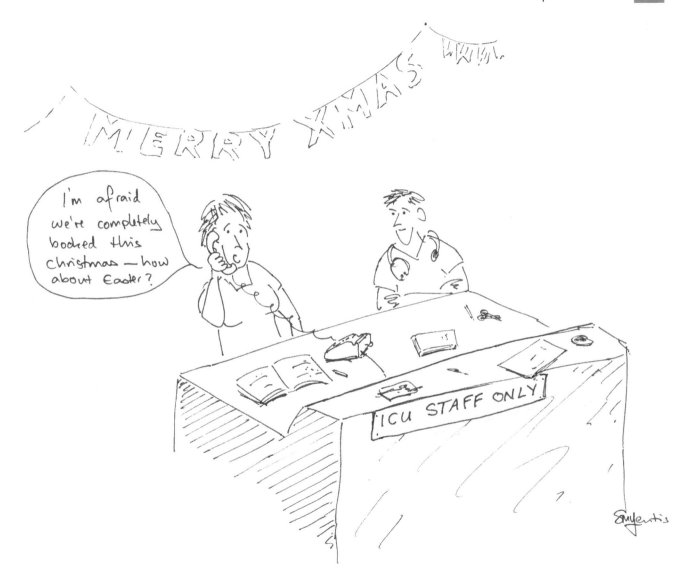

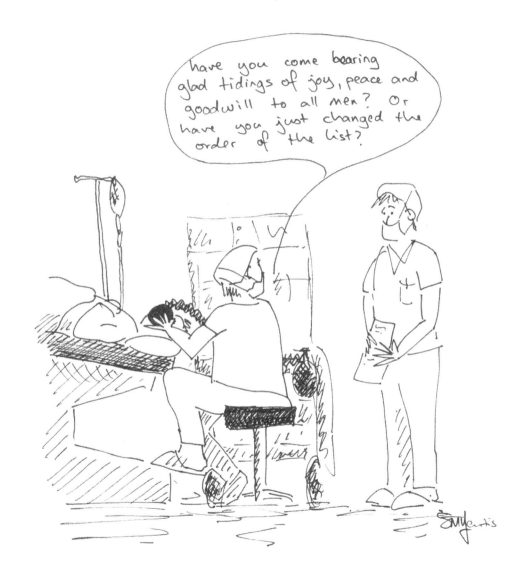

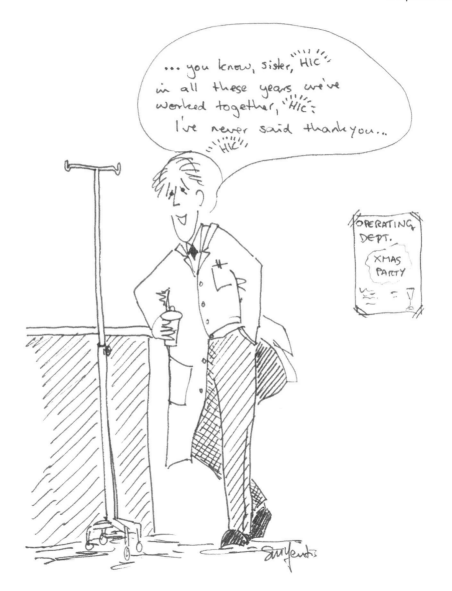

Chapter 9

The boundaries of knowledge

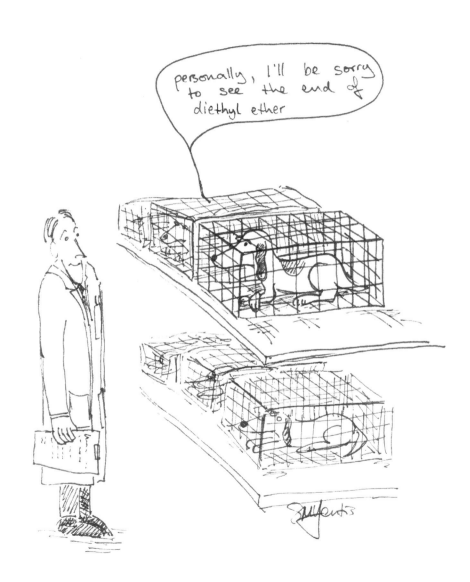

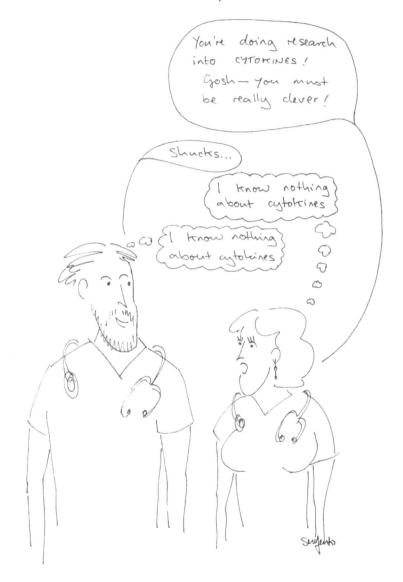

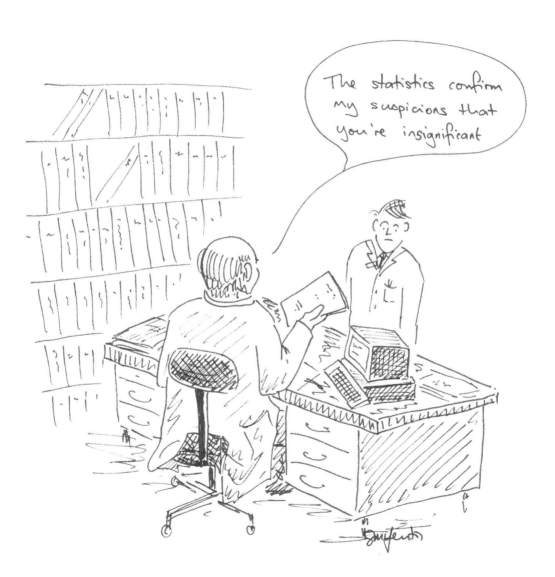

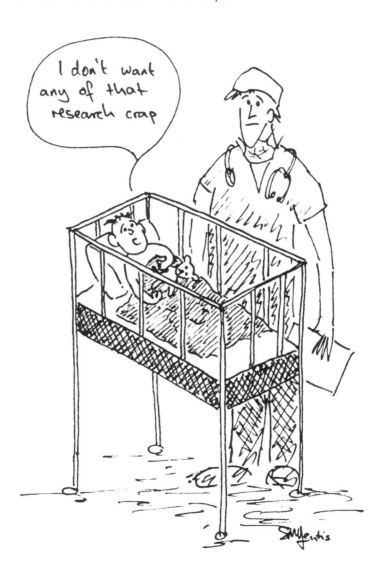

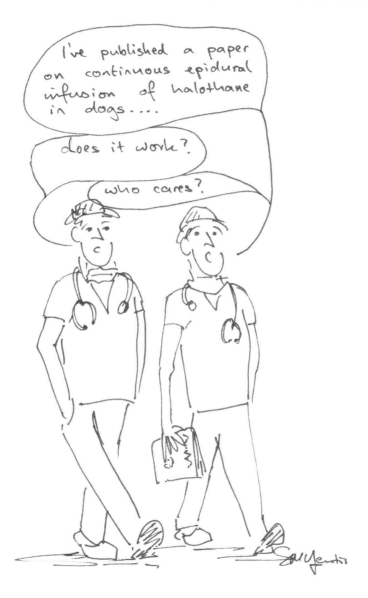

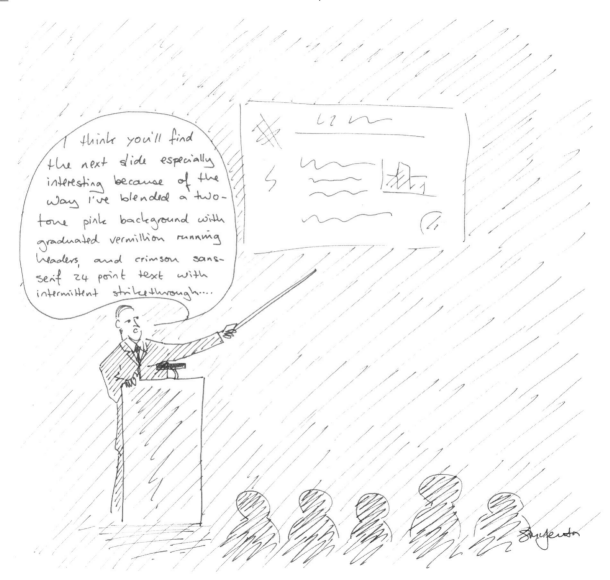

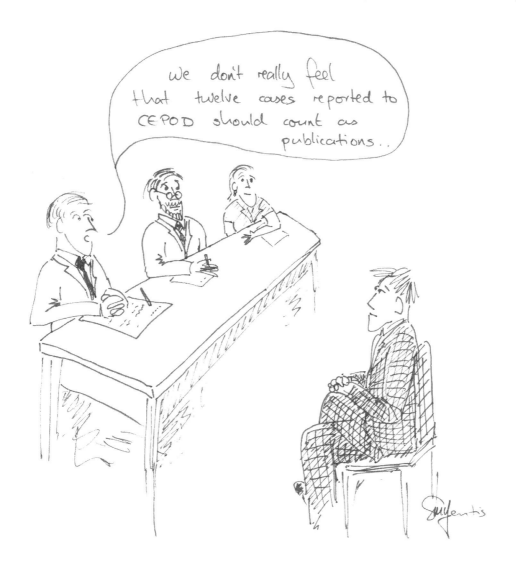

Chapter 10

Painful clinics

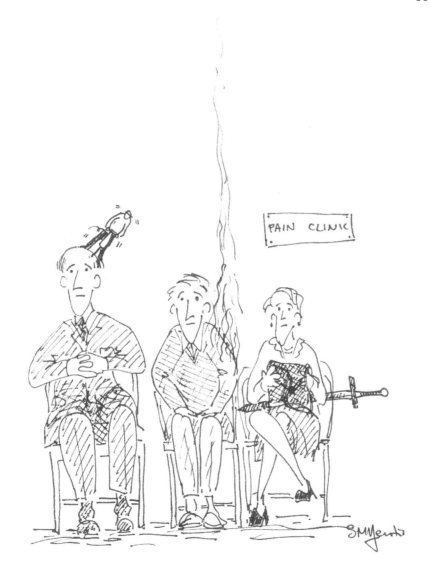

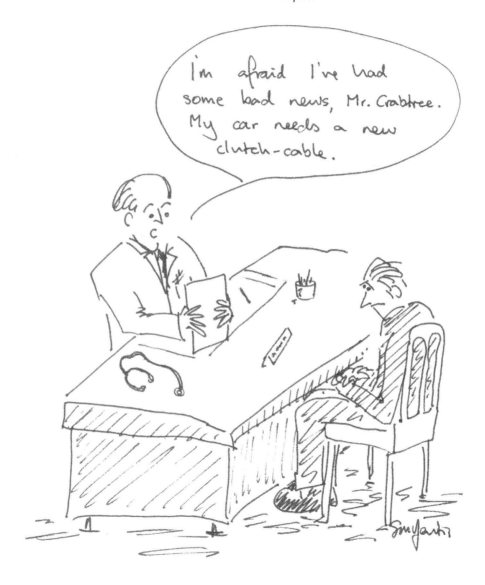

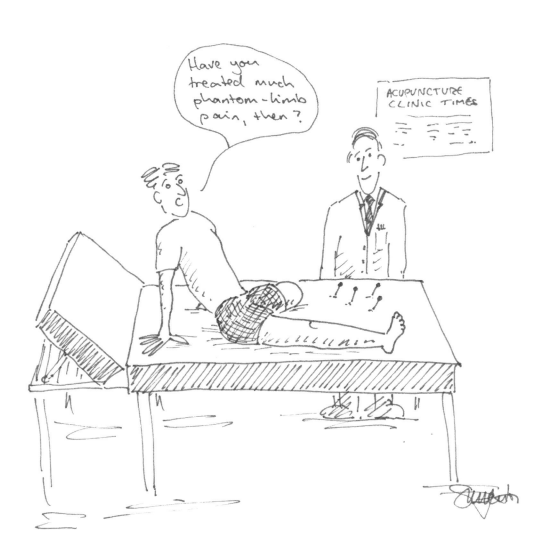

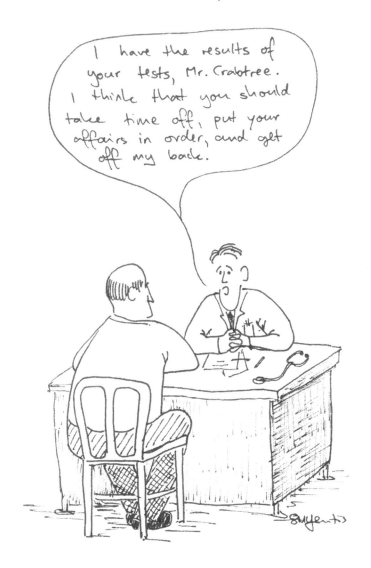

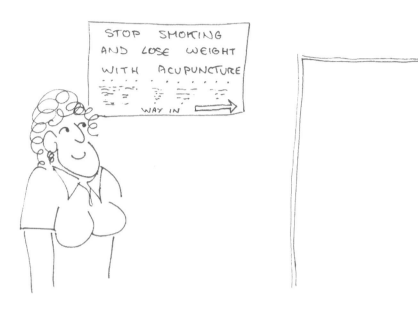
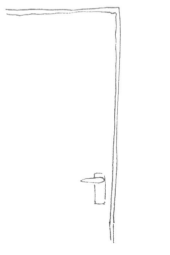
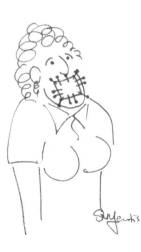

Chapter 11

Passing the exam

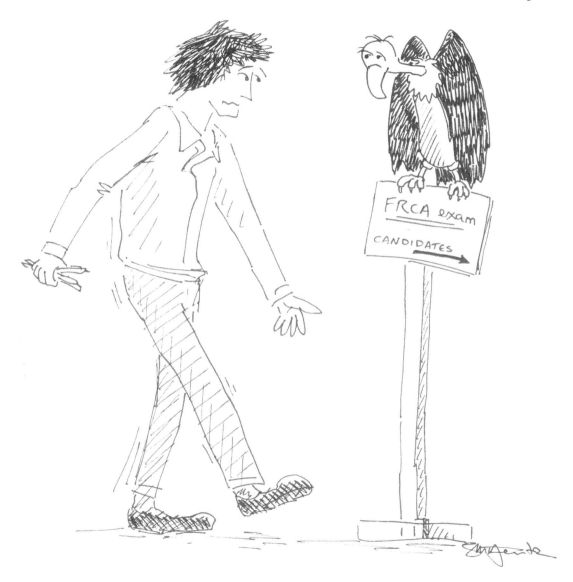

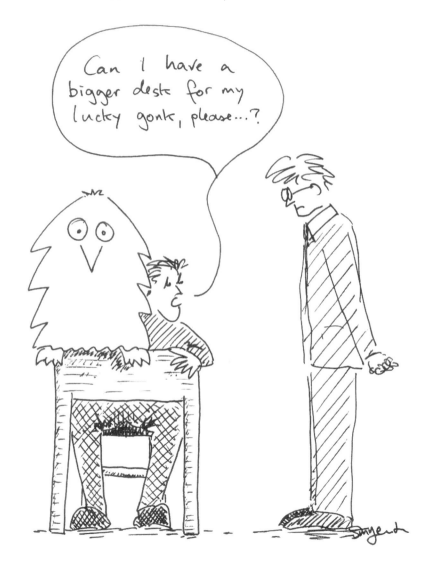

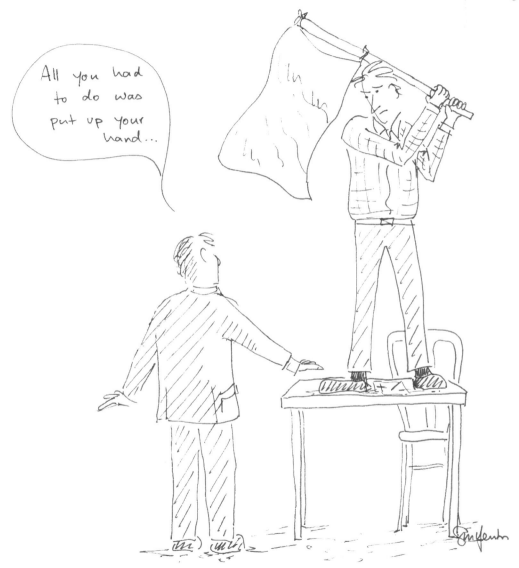

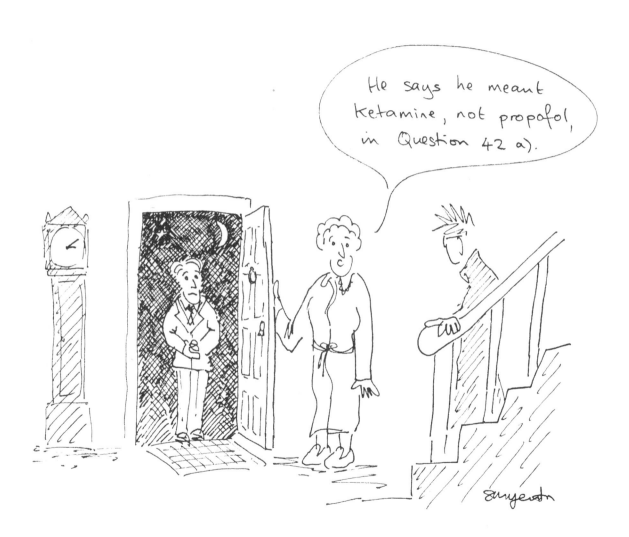

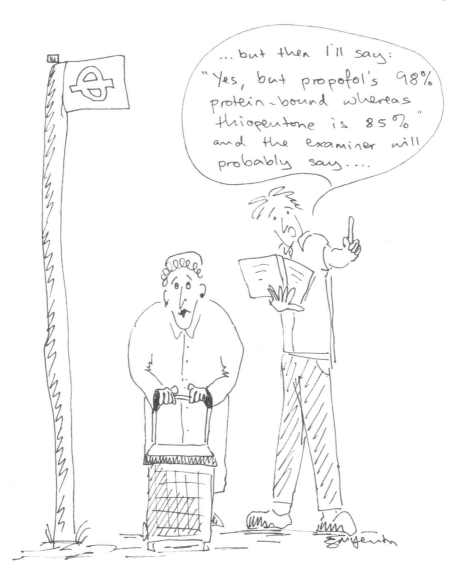

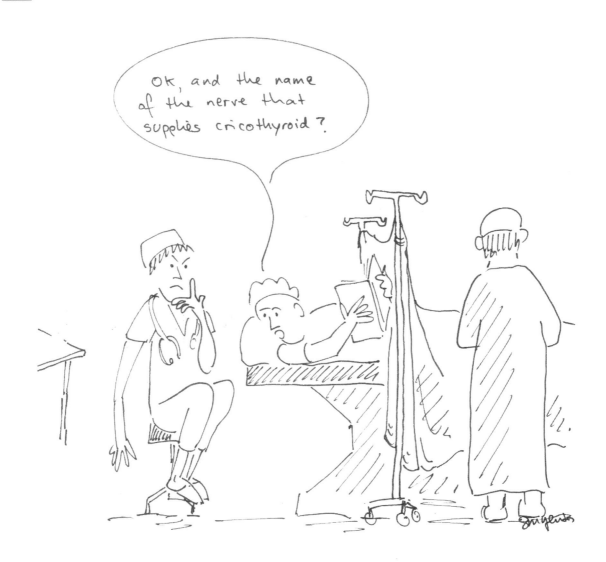

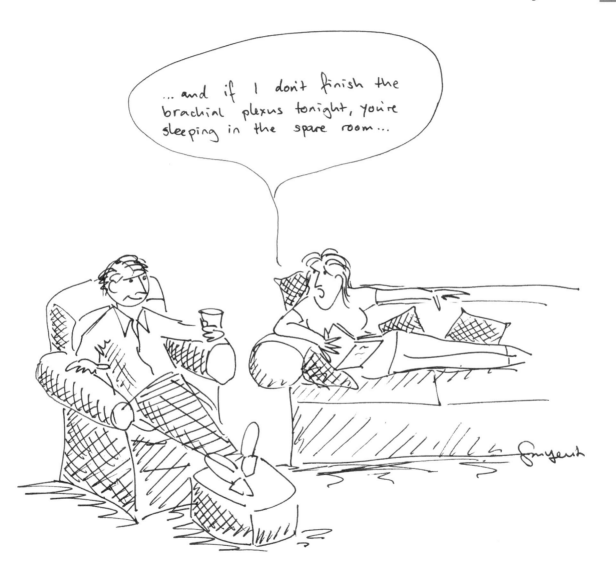

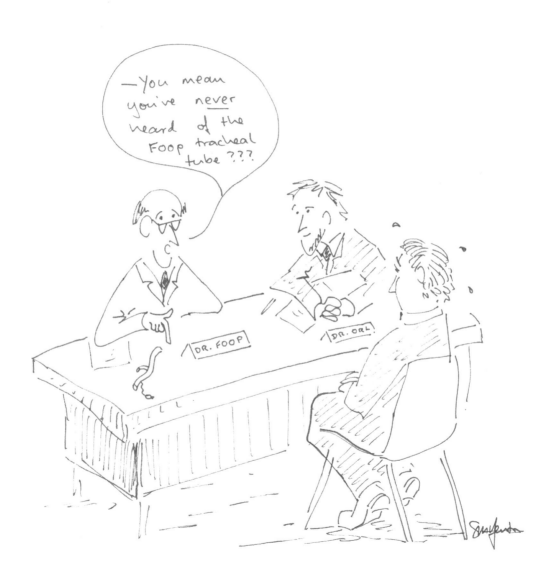

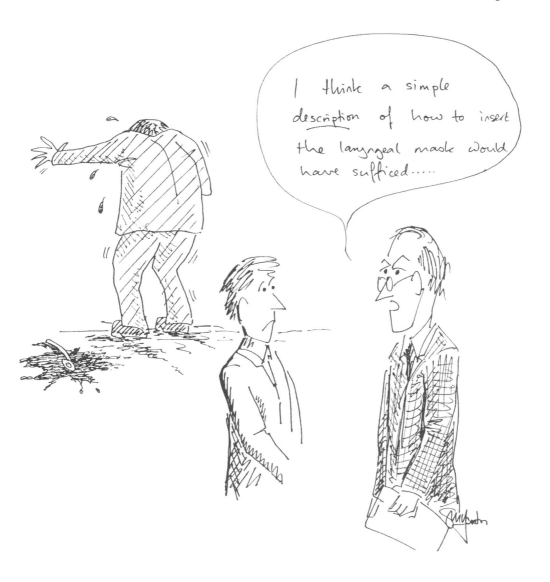

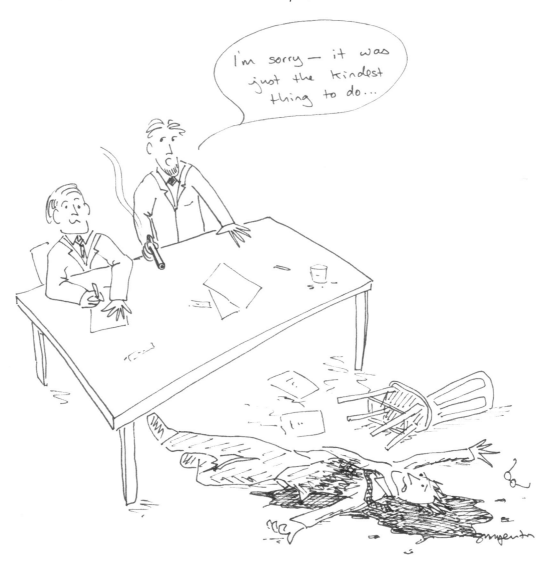

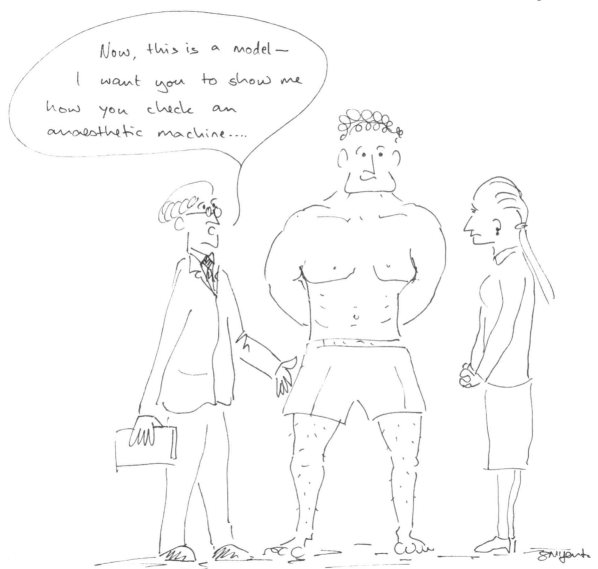

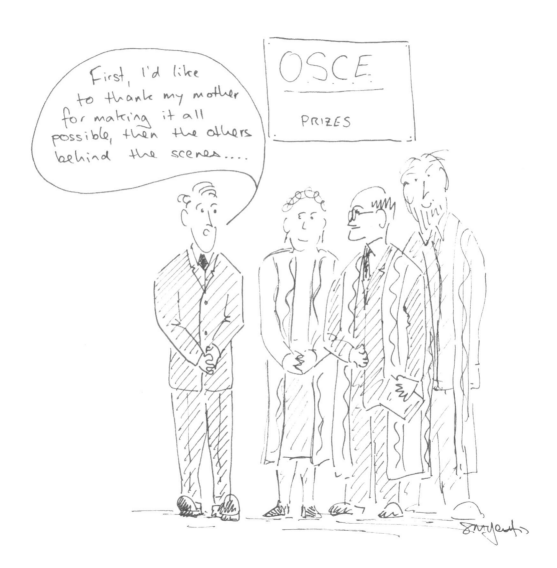

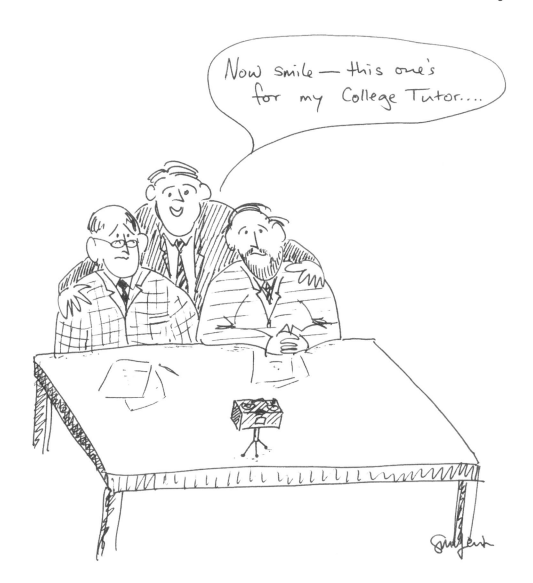

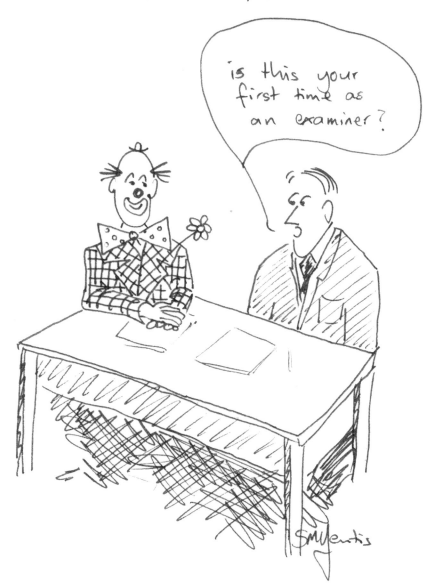

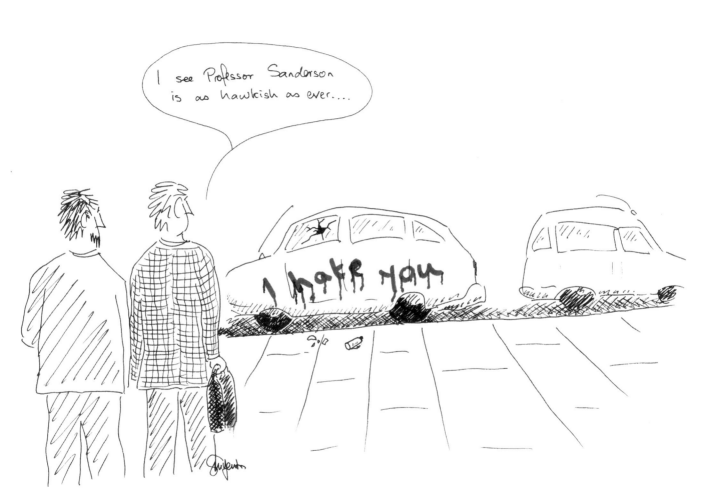

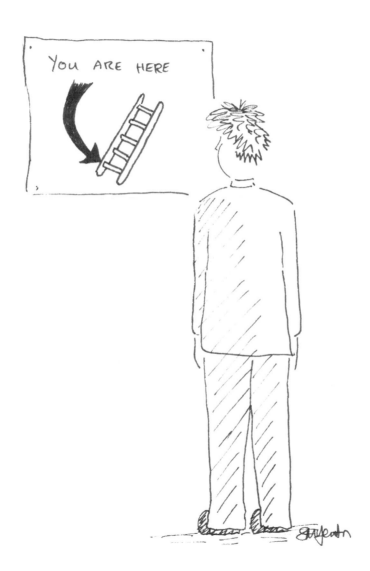

Chapter 12

Pot-pourri

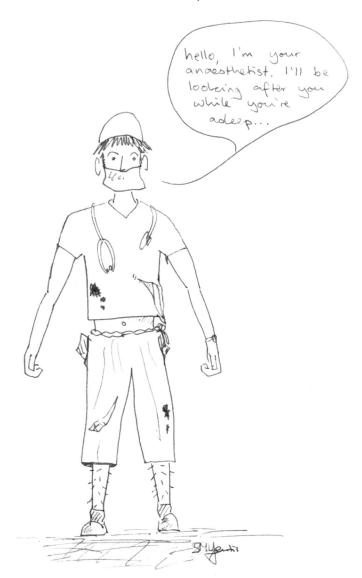

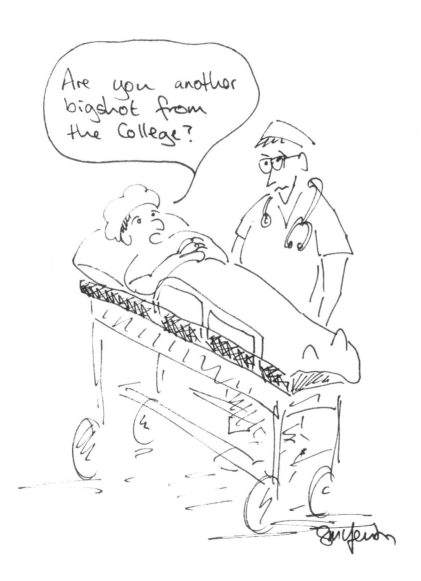

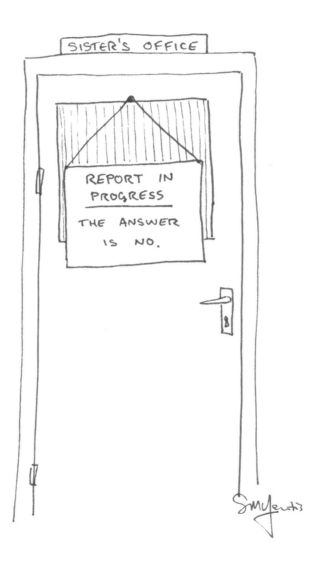

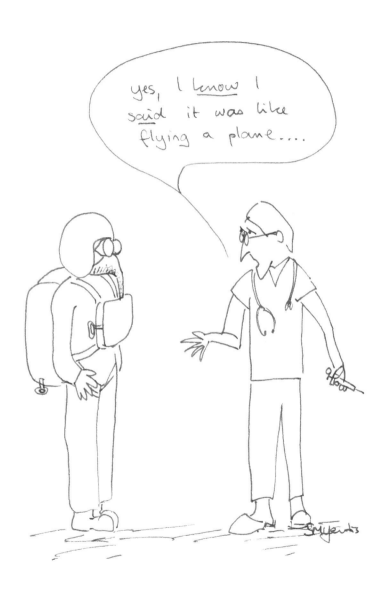

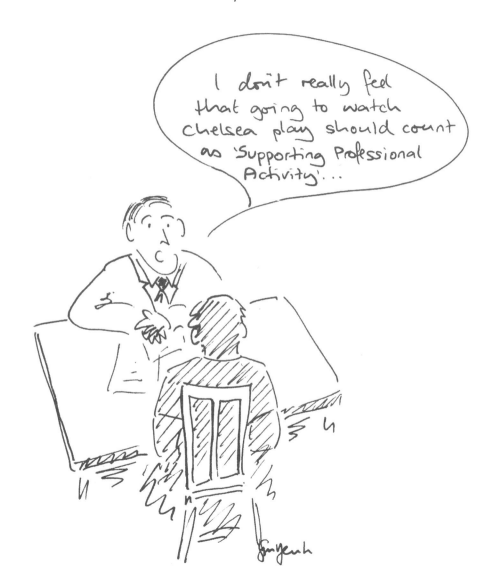

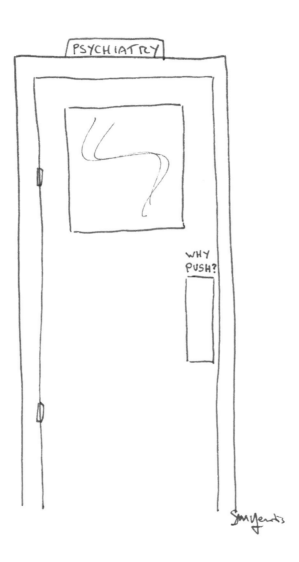

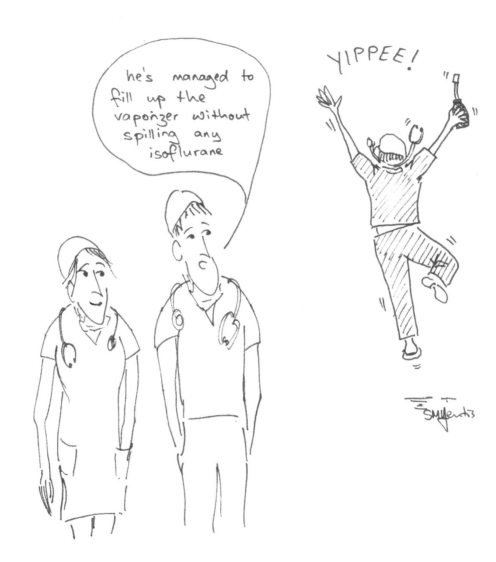

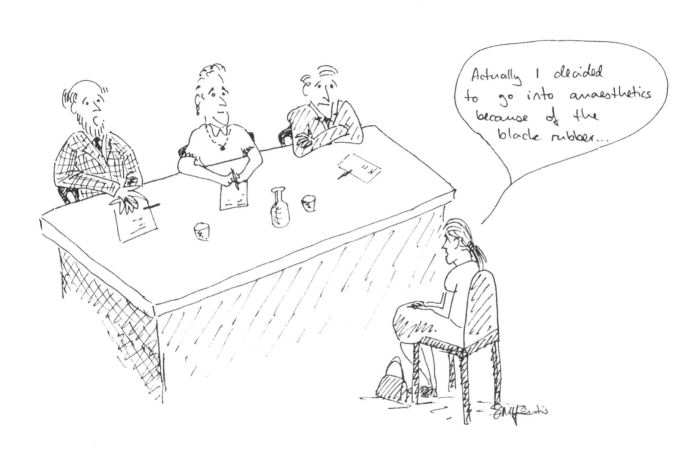

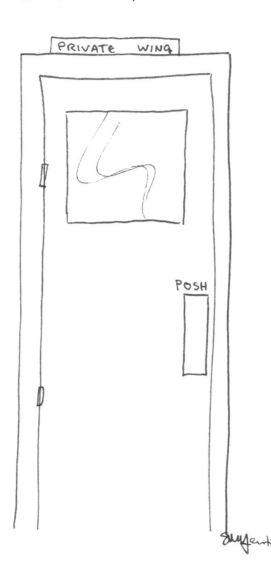

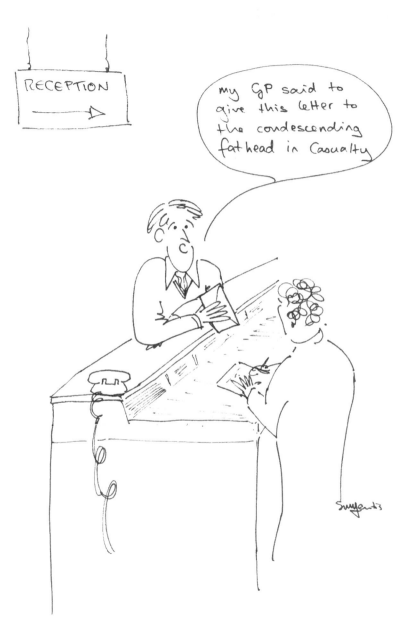

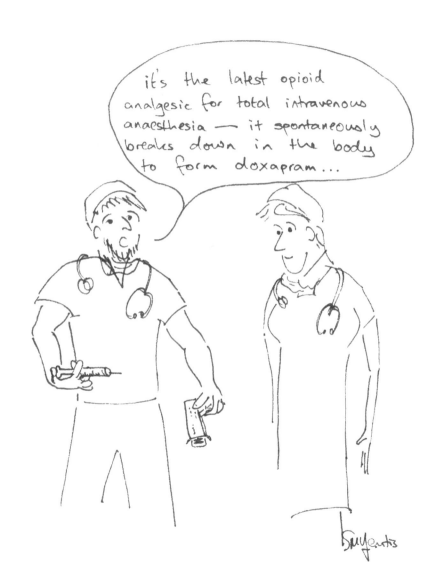

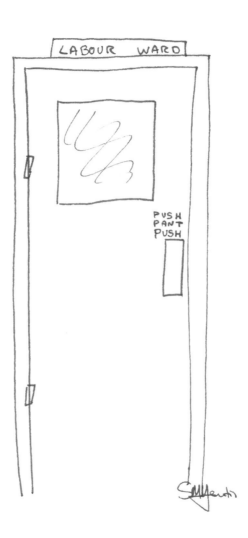

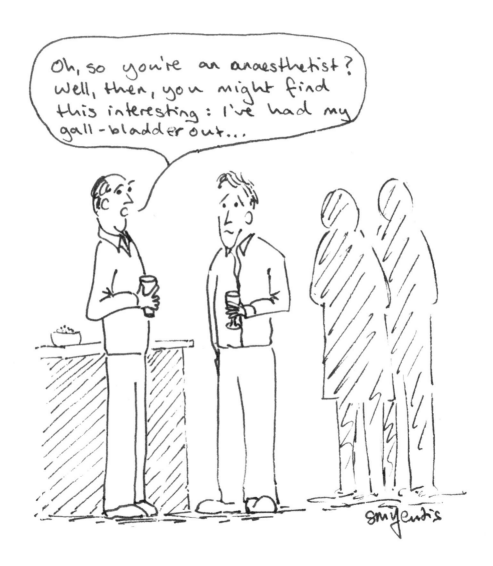

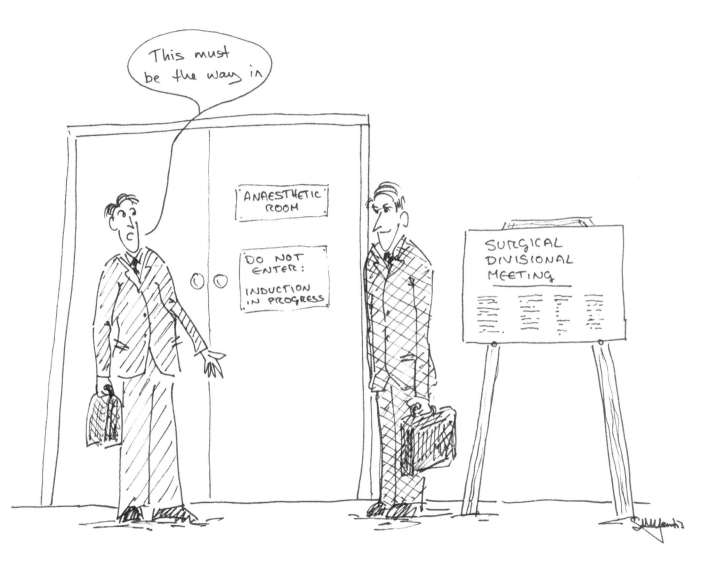

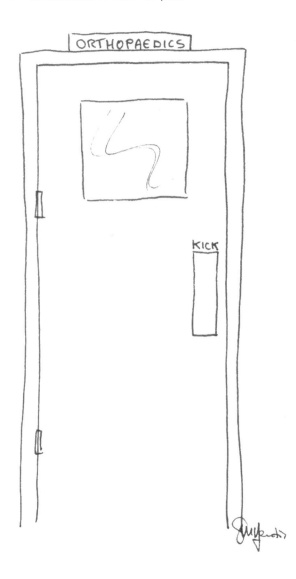

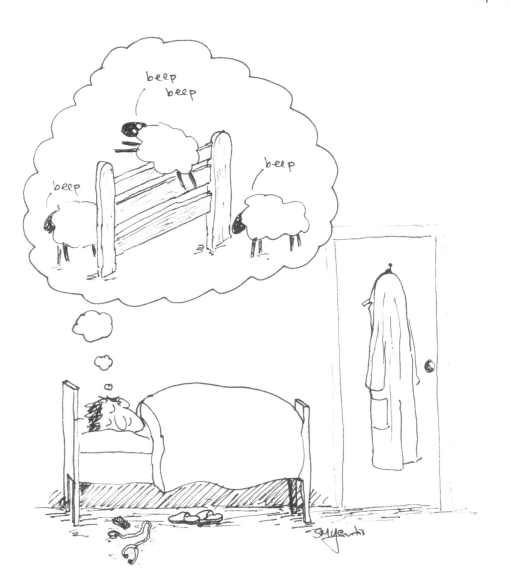

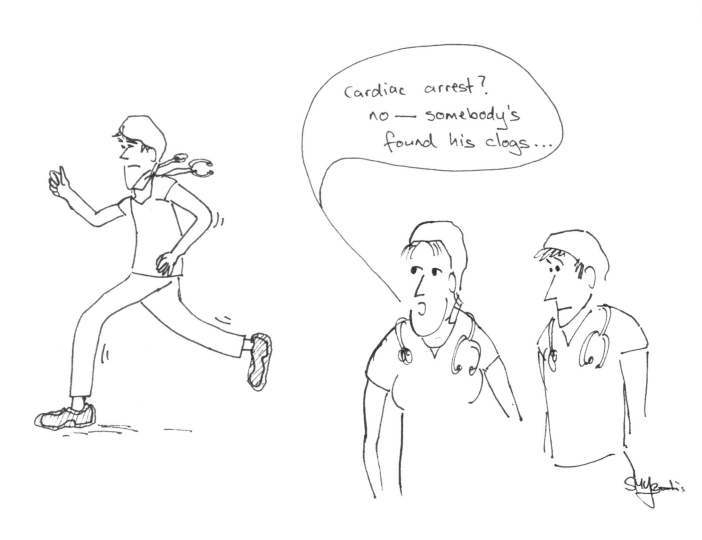

THE SURGEON AT HOME

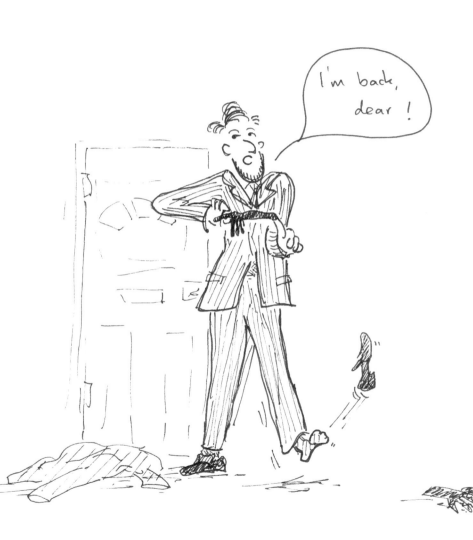

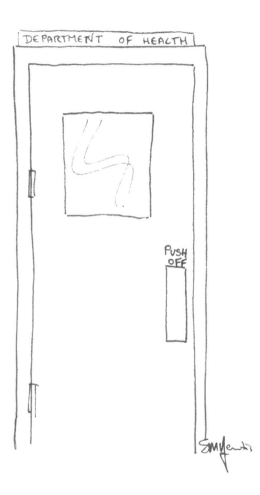